REBECCA PARK TOTILO

Natural Acne Treatment

WITH ESSENTIAL OIL

Natural Acne Treatment with Essential Oil

Copyright © 2024 by Rebecca Park Totilo
All rights reserved. No part of this book may be reproduced or transmitted in any form or by any means without the author's written permission.

Printed in the United States of America.
Published by Rebecca at the Well Foundation.

No part of this publication may be reproduced, stored in a retrieval system, or transmitted in any form by any means—electronic, mechanical, photocopy, recording, or otherwise—without written permission of the copyright holder, except as provided by USA copyright law.

Disclaimer Notice: The information contained in this book is intended for educational purposes only and is not meant to substitute for medical care or prescribe treatment for any specific health condition. Please see a qualified healthcare provider for medical treatment. The author and publisher assume no responsibility or liability for any person or group for any loss, damage, or injury resulting from using or misusing any information in this book. No express or implied guarantee is given regarding the effects of using any of the products described herein.

Paperback ISBN: 979-8-9872464-4-3
Electronic ISBN: 979-8-9872464-6-7

Table of Contents

Introduction 1

Chapter 1: Understanding Acne 3
- What Is Acne? 3
- Causes of Acne 4
- The Development of Acne 4
- Types of Acne 5
- Severity of Acne 5
- Gender Differences in Acne 6
- Seeking Help 6

Chapter 2: Types of Acne 7
- Whiteheads 7
- Blackheads 8
- Papules 9
- Pustules 9
- Nodules 10
- Cysts 10
- Acne Severity 11
- Conclusion 11

Chapter 3: Stages of Acne 13
- Mild Acne 13
- Moderate Acne 14
- Severe Acne 15
- Gender Differences in Acne Severity 16
- Seeking Professional Help 16
- Conclusion 17

Chapter 4: Acne Myths and Truths 19
- Myth 1: Stress Causes Acne 20
- Myth 2: Eating Chocolate and Greasy Foods Causes Acne 20
- Myth 3: Dirty Skin Causes Acne 21
- Myth 4: Sun Exposure Clears Up Acne 21
- Myth 5: Popping Pimples Helps Them Heal Faster 22
- Myth 6: Only Teenagers Get Acne 22
- Myth 7: Makeup Causes Acne 23
- Myth 8: Acne Is Contagious 23
- Myth 9: You'll Outgrow Acne, So Leave It Alone 24

- Myth 10: Sweating Helps Clean Out Hair Follicle Areas 24
- Myth 11: Acne Problems Are Directly Proportionate to Sexual Activity 25
- Myth 12: People with Acne Are Dirty and Don't Wash Enough 25
- Myth 13: Acne Is Only a Surface Issue 26
- Myth 14: There Is a Cure for Acne 26
- Myth 15: Certain Cosmetics or Spot Treatments Will Help Acne 27
- Myth 16: People with Acne Should Not Use Moisturizers or Makeup 27
- Conclusion 28

Chapter 5: Skin Care and Acne Prevention 29
- Exercise 30
- Cosmetics 30
- Diet 31
- Hormones 32
- Hygiene 32
- Products 32
- Shaving 33
- Stress 33

Chapter 6: Treatment with Essential Oils 35
- Timing and Approach 36
- Proactiv Solution 36
- Essential Oil Acne Treatment System 37
- Supplemental Products 39

Chapter 7: Essential Oils for Skin Rejuvenation 43
- Skin Regeneration and Youthfulness 44
- Improving Muscle Tone and Blood Circulation 44
- Supporting the Skin's Protective Barrier 45
- Anti-Inflammatory Properties 45
- Balancing Sebum Production 45
- Incorporating Essential Oils into Skincare Products 46
- Recommended Essential Oils for Acne 46
- Essential Oils for Skin Infection and Deodorization 47

Chapter 8: Carrier Oils 49
- Tamanu Oil 50
- Jojoba Oil 50
- Grapeseed Oil 51
- Argan Oil 51
- Rosehip Seed Oil 52
- Calendula Oil 52
- Hemp Seed Oil 52

Chapter 9: Essential Oils for Acne 53
- Acne 54
- Astringent 55
- Blackheads and Pimples 56
- Scars 57
- Inflammation 57

Chapter 10: Facial Masks 59
- Tea Tree and Honey Facial Mask 60
- Bentonite Clay and Lemon Mask 61
- Charcoal and Eucalyptus Mask 62
- Yogurt and Peppermint Face Mask 63
- Aloe Vera and Clove Bud Mask 64
- Cucumber and Chamomile Refreshing Mask 65
- Tea Tree and Bentonite Clay Mask 66
- Neem and Turmeric Mask 67
- Ginger and Green Tea Mask 68
- Yogurt and Sandalwood Mask 69
- Tea Tree and Lavender Overnight Mask 70
- Chamomile and Honey Overnight Mask 71
- Frankincense and Rose Water Overnight Mask 72
- Peppermint and Green Tea Overnight Mask 73
- Rosemary and Clay Overnight Mask 74

Chapter 11: Exfoliating Scrubs 75
- Lavender and Oatmeal Scrub 76
- Tea Tree and Coconut Scrub 77
- Lemon and Honey Exfoliating Mask 78
- Green Tea and Matcha Scrub 79
- Aloe Vera and Rose Scrub 80
- Bentonite Clay and Lavender Cream 81
- Mint and Sea Salt Scrub 82
- Oatmeal and Tea Tree Exfoliating Cream 83
- Honey and Lemon Sugar Scrub 84
- Coconut and Activated Charcoal Scrub 85

Chapter 12: Facial Cleansers 87
- Jojoba and Green Tea Facial Cleanser 89
- Tea Tree Foaming Cleanser 90
- Aloe Vera and Chamomile Cleanser 91
- Honey and Lemon Cleanser 92
- Green Tea and Peppermint Cleanser 93
- Yogurt and Honey Cleanser 94
- Coconut Oil and Frankincense Cleanser 95

- Rose Water and Jojoba Cleanser 96
- Apple Cider Vinegar and Tea Tree Cleanser 97
- Bentonite Clay and Lavender Cleanser 98
- Gentle Tea Tree Cleanser 99
- Clarifying Lemon Cleanser 100
- Purifying Charcoal Cleanser 101
- Calming Chamomile Cleanser 102
- Soothing Aloe Cleanser 103
- Refreshing Peppermint Cleanser 104
- Hydrating Coconut Cleanser 105
- Detoxifying Green Tea Cleanser 106
- Gentle Rose Cleanser 107
- Brightening Citrus Cleanser 108

Chapter 13: Spot Treatments 109

- Honey and Cinnamon Spot Treatment 111
- Tea Tree Spot Treatment 112
- Lavender and Frankincense Spot Treatment 113
- Peppermint and Lemon Spot Treatment 114
- Green Tea and Tea Tree Spot Treatment 115
- Benzoyl Peroxide and Eucalyptus Spot Treatment 116
- Clove Bud and Geranium Spot Treatment 117
- Chamomile and Rosehip Seed Oil Spot Treatment 118
- Myrrh and Witch Hazel Spot Treatment 119
- Carrot Seed and Lavender Spot Treatment 120

Chapter 14: Serums 121

- Rosehip and Green Tea Serum 123
- Tea Tree and Jojoba Serum 124
- Frankincense and Argan Serum 125
- Rosehip and Chamomile Serum 126
- Lavender and Grapeseed Serum 127
- Aloe Vera and Sandalwood Serum 128
- Clary Sage and Hemp Seed Serum 129
- Calendula and Neroli Serum 130
- Tamanu and Geranium Serum 131
- Neem and Rosemary Serum 132
- Balancing Acne Serum 133
- Hydrating Acne Serum 134
- Clarifying Anti-Acne Serum 135
- Soothing Redness Serum 136
- Anti-Inflammatory Acne Serum 137
- Nourishing Night Serum 138
- Brightening Acne Serum 139

- Blemish-Fighting Serum 140
- Skin-Balancing Serum 141
- Healing Acne Scar Serum 142
- Gentle Acne Serum 143

Chapter 15: Roll-On Recipes 145

- Acne Spot Treatment Roll-On 147
- Soothing Anti-Acne Roll-On 148
- Calming Lavender and Tea Tree Roll-On 149
- Clary Sage and Geranium Acne Roll-On 150
- Purifying Lemongrass and Peppermint Roll-On 151
- Healing Rosehip and Myrrh Roll-On 152
- Brightening Lemon and Carrot Seed Roll-On 153
- Soothing Chamomile and Sandalwood Roll-On 154
- Blemish-Fighting Oregano and Tea Tree Roll-On 155
- Anti-Redness Frankincense and Lavender Roll-On 156

Chapter 16: Body Cleanser Recipes 157

- Gentle Tea Tree Cleanser 159
- Clarifying Lemon Cleanser 160
- Balancing Geranium Cleanser 161
- Revitalizing Peppermint Cleanser 162
- Soothing Chamomile Cleanser 163
- Detoxifying Charcoal Cleanser 164
- Calming Aloe and Lavender Cleanser 165
- Brightening Citrus Cleanser 166
- Exfoliating Oat and Lavender Cleanser 167
- Nourishing Honey and Almond Cleanser 168
- Hydrating Rose and Aloe Cleanser 169

Chapter 17: Facial Mists and Spray Recipes 171

- Acne-Fighting Facial Mist 173
- Refreshing Antibacterial Spray 174
- Calming Facial Toner Spray 175
- Purifying Detox Spray 176
- Aloe Vera and Rose Water Face Mist 177
- Green Tea and Cucumber Face Mist 178
- Rose Water and Chamomile Face Mist 179
- Green Tea and Mint Face Mist 180
- Rose Water and Witch Hazel Face Mist 181
- Aloe Vera and Green Tea Face Mist 182

Chapter 18: Makeup Remover Pads 183

- Gentle Makeup Remover Pads 184

- Refreshing Citrus Makeup Remover Pads 185
- Calming Rose Water Makeup Remover Pads 186
- Hydrating Makeup Remover Pads 187
- Detoxifying Green Tea Makeup Remover Pads 188
- Soothing Aloe and Cucumber Makeup Remover Pads 189
- Anti-Inflammatory Calendula Makeup Remover Pads 190
- Brightening Neroli Makeup Remover Pads 191
- Clarifying Mint and Lemon Makeup Remover Pads 192
- Deep Cleansing Charcoal Makeup Remover Pads 193

Chapter 19: Milk Baths 195

- Rose and Lime Milk Bath 196
- Lavender and Oatmeal Milk Bath 197
- Tea Tree and Epsom Salt Milk Bath 198
- Chamomile and Honey Milk Bath 199
- Rosemary and Sea Salt Milk Bath 200
- Peppermint and Green Tea Milk Bath 201
- Lemongrass and Coconut Milk Bath 202
- Frankincense and Almond Milk Bath 203
- Geranium and Rose Milk Bath 204
- Orange and Calendula Milk Bath 205

Chapter 20: Acne Patches 207

- Tea Tree and Aloe Vera Patch 208
- Lavender and Witch Hazel Patch 209
- Frankincense and Chamomile Patch 210
- Clary Sage and Rose Water Patch 211
- Lemon and Honey Patch 212
- Peppermint and Green Tea Patch 213
- Geranium and Apple Cider Vinegar Patch 214
- Eucalyptus and Aloe Vera Patch 215
- Tea Tree and Jojoba Oil Patch 216
- Rosemary and Witch Hazel Patch 217

Chapter 21: Toners for Acne 219

- Tea Tree and Witch Hazel Toner 220
- Rose Water and Aloe Toner 221
- Apple Cider Vinegar and Lavender Toner 222
- Green Tea and Chamomile Toner 223
- Cucumber and Rose Water Toner 224
- Aloe and Rosemary Toner 225
- Mint and Lemon Toner 226
- Orange Blossom and Neroli Toner 227
- Witch Hazel and Basil Toner 228

- Cypress and Rose Water Toner 229

Chapter 22: Moisturizers for Acne 231

- Unscented Lotion Base 232
- Tea Tree and Lavender Moisturizer 233
- Aloe and Frankincense Soothing Moisturizer 234
- Mattifying Moisturizer with Geranium and Clary Sage 235
- Rosehip and Tea Tree Night Moisturizer 236
- Hydrating Moisturizer with Rose and Chamomile 237
- Green Tea and Aloe Moisturizer 238
- Chamomile and Calendula Calming Moisturizer 239
- Neem and Lavender Moisturizer 240
- Aloe Vera and Rosehip Moisturizer 241

Chapter 23: Essential Oil Directory 243

- Angelica (Angelica archangelica) 245
- Bay (Pimenta racemosa) 245
- Bay Laurel (Laurus nobilis) 245
- Basil (Ocimum basilicum) 246
- Benzoin (Styrax benzoin) 246
- Bergamot (Citrus bergamia) 247
- Birch (Betula lenta) 247
- Camphor (Cinnamomum camphora) 247
- Cajeput (Melaleuca cajuputi) 248
- Caraway Seed (Carum carvi) 248
- Carrot Seed (Daucus carota) 249
- Cedarwood (Cedrus atlantica) 249
- German Chamomile (Matricaria chamomilla) 249
- Roman Chamomile (Chamaemelum nobile) 250
- Cinnamon (Cinnamomum zeylanicum) 250
- Cistus Labdanum (Cistus ladaniferus) 251
- Citronella (Cymbopogon nardus) 251
- Clary Sage (Salvia sclarea) 251
- Clove Bud (Syzygium aromaticum) 252
- Coriander (Coriandrum sativum) 252
- Cypress (Cupressus sempervirens) 253
- Eucalyptus (Eucalyptus globulus) 253
- Fleabane (Erigeron canadensis) 253
- Frankincense (Boswellia carterii) 254
- Galbanum (Ferula galbaniflua) 254
- Geranium (Pelargonium graveolens) 255
- Grapefruit (Citrus paradisi) 255
- Helichrysum (Helichrysum italicum) 256
- Hyssop (Hyssopus officinalis) 256

- ❖ Jasmine (Jasminum officinale) 256
- ❖ Juniper Berry (Juniperus communis) 257
- ❖ Lavender (Lavandula angustifolia) 257
- ❖ Lemon (Citrus limon) 258
- ❖ Lemon Myrtle (Backhousia citriodora) 258
- ❖ Lemongrass (Cymbopogon citratus) 259
- ❖ Lime (Citrus aurantiifolia) 259
- ❖ Linaloe Berry (Bursera delpechiana) 260
- ❖ Mandarin (Citrus reticulata) 260
- ❖ May Chang (Litsea cubeba) 260
- ❖ Melissa (Melissa officinalis) 261
- ❖ Myrrh (Commiphora myrrha) 261
- ❖ Myrtle (Myrtus communis) 262
- ❖ Neroli (Citrus aurantium var. amara) 262
- ❖ Niaouli (Melaleuca quinquenervia) 262
- ❖ Opoponax (Commiphora erythraea) 263
- ❖ Orange (Citrus sinensis) 263
- ❖ Oregano (Origanum vulgare) 264
- ❖ Palmarosa (Cymbopogon martinii) 264
- ❖ Parsley (Petroselinum crispum) 265
- ❖ Patchouli (Pogostemon cablin) 265
- ❖ Peppermint (Mentha piperita) 265
- ❖ Petitgrain (Citrus aurantium var. amara) 266
- ❖ Plai (Zingiber cassumunar) 266
- ❖ Rose (Rosa damascena) 267
- ❖ Rose Geranium (Pelargonium graveolens) 267
- ❖ Rosemary (Rosmarinus officinalis) 268
- ❖ Rosewood (Aniba rosaeodora) 268
- ❖ Sage (Salvia officinalis) 269
- ❖ Sandalwood (Santalum album) 269
- ❖ Spearmint (Mentha spicata) 269
- ❖ Spikenard (Nardostachys jatamansi) 270
- ❖ Spruce (Picea mariana) 270
- ❖ Tarragon (Artemisia dracunculus) 271
- ❖ Tea Tree (Melaleuca alternifolia) 271
- ❖ Thyme (Thymus vulgaris) 271
- ❖ Vetiver (Vetiveria zizanioides) 272
- ❖ Violet (Viola odorata) 272
- ❖ Yarrow (Achillea millefolium) 272
- ❖ Ylang Ylang (Cananga odorata) 273

Other Books by Rebecca Park Totilo 275

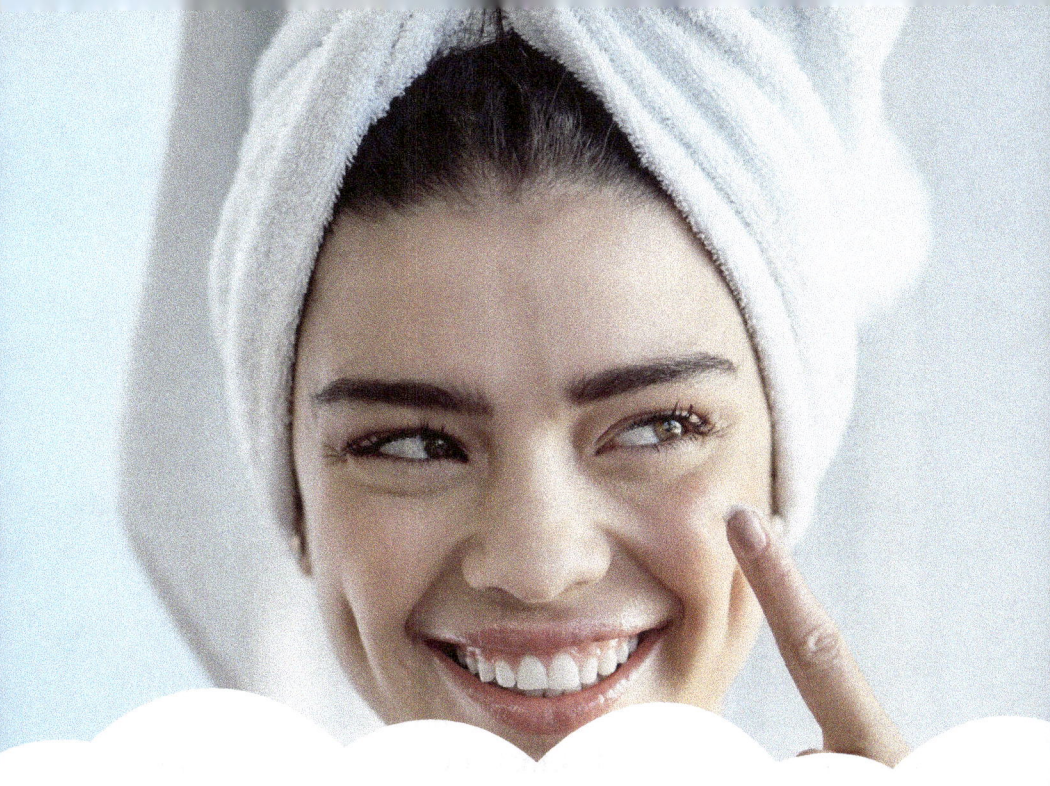

Introduction

Acne is a pervasive issue affecting a significant portion of the population, with reports indicating that over 90% of adolescents and nearly 25% of adults suffer from this condition. Acne can impact one's appearance, self-esteem, and overall quality of life. Understanding its causes and finding effective treatments is crucial for those affected.

In this book, we will explore acne comprehensively, aiming to clear up common myths and misconceptions about its causes. For example, does indulging in chocolate lead to breakouts? Are oily foods like French fries to blame for acne flare-ups? We will uncover the facts behind these questions by examining the most recent studies, reports, and articles.

Moreover, this book will focus on the potential benefits of essential oils in treating and preventing acne. Essential oils have been used for centuries for their therapeutic properties, and recent research suggests they may play a significant role in skin care. We will explore which essential oils can help minimize acne outbreaks, reduce inflammation, and nourish the skin, providing natural and holistic options for managing this common skin condition.

It's important to note that the content presented here is for educational purposes and is not a substitute for professional medical advice. Remember that any healthcare decisions should be made with your medical and health professionals. This book aims to provide an overview of current acne research and potential natural remedies, empowering you to make informed decisions about your skin care.

Join us as we delve into the complexities of acne, debunk myths, and discover the potential of essential oils in promoting clear and healthy skin.

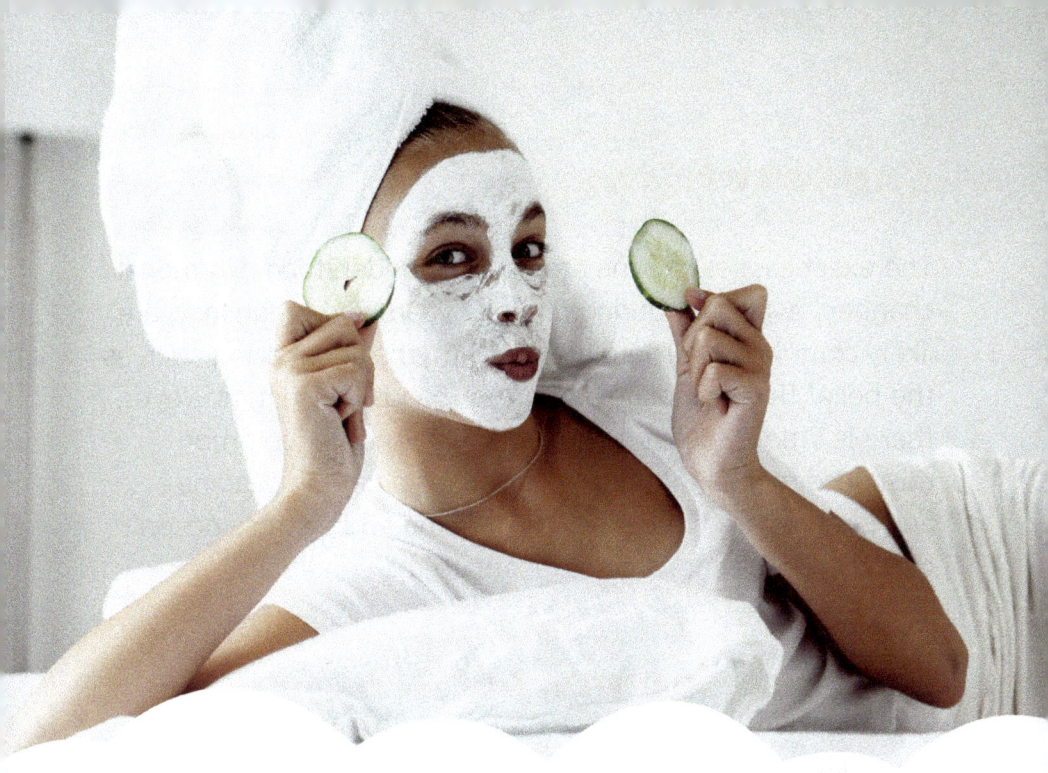

Chapter 1
Understanding Acne

What Is Acne?

Acne is a common skin condition that results in pimples. Pimples form when hair follicles under the skin become clogged. Acne often appears on the face, neck, back, chest, and shoulders. While anyone can develop acne, it is prevalent among teenagers and young adults. Though not usually severe, acne can lead to scarring.

Causes of Acne

The exact causes of acne are not fully understood. Hormonal changes, especially during teenage years and pregnancy, are likely contributors. There are many myths about acne, such as the belief that chocolate and greasy foods cause it; however, there is little evidence to support this. Another common misconception is that dirty skin causes acne. Blackheads and pimples are not caused by dirt, and while stress doesn't directly cause acne, it can exacerbate the condition.

The Development of Acne

Acne develops through a few key steps:

Clogged Pores: Hair follicles, or pores, become blocked for various reasons. Contributing factors include genetics, hormones, diet, vitamin deficiencies, and stress. Environmental factors, overall health, and hormonal influences on sebum production also play a role.

Blocked Pores: Dead skin cells and sebum (natural skin oil) combine and become trapped in these blocked pores, creating a sticky substance that further clogs the passage.

Bacterial Growth: Bacteria begin to grow in the clogged areas. The body's white blood cells respond by attacking the bacteria, leading to inflammation as they attempt to expel the bacteria.

Formation of Microcomedones: This battle results in microcomedones, which can develop into visible blemishes known as comedones or, more commonly, pimples or acne.

Types of Acne

Acne can manifest in various forms, each with its own characteristics. The four main types of acne are:

- **Whiteheads:** When sebum and bacteria are trapped beneath the skin's surface, forming a visible white bump.
- **Blackheads:** When sebum and bacteria are only partially trapped, draining slowly to the surface and turning black due to exposure to air and skin's melanin.
- **Pimples:** General term for smaller inflamed lesions without a clear head.
- **Nodules:** Deeper, boil-like lesions that can be painful and more challenging to treat.

For a more detailed exploration of the different types of acne, see Chapter 2.

Severity of Acne

Acne can range from mild to severe:

- **Mild Acne:** Characterized by whiteheads and blackheads, and occasionally pimples.
- **Moderate Acne:** Includes more pimples and blemishes, possibly spreading to the back or chest.

- **Severe Acne:** Features many large, painful nodules on the face, back, chest, and other areas. This type often leads to scarring.

Gender Differences in Acne

Males often experience more severe acne due to hormonal differences. They tend to develop acne in areas like the chest and back, which can be more difficult to treat.

Seeking Help

For those with potential nodular acne or severe cases, seeking advice from a healthcare provider is recommended to prevent scarring and manage the condition effectively.

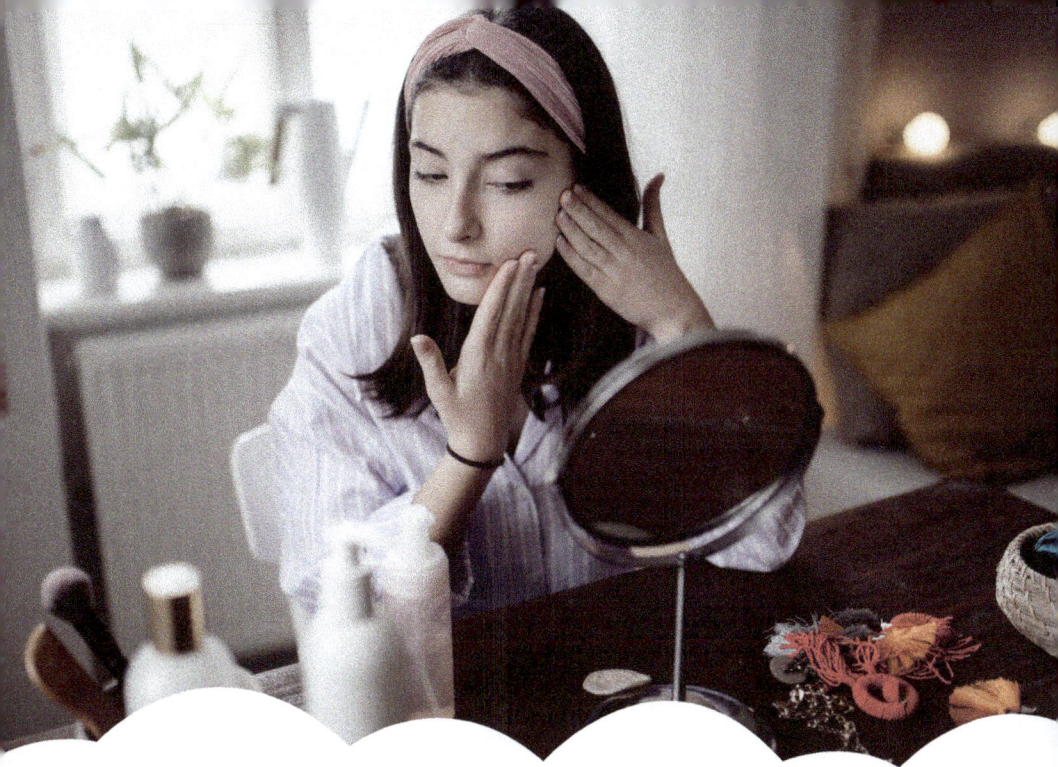

Chapter 2
Types of Acne

Acne can manifest in various forms, each with its own characteristics and treatment considerations. Understanding the different types of acne is essential for effective management and treatment. This chapter will explore the primary types of acne, their features, and how they develop.

Whiteheads

Whiteheads are a type of acne that occurs when sebum (natural skin oil) and dead skin cells become trapped beneath the skin's surface. This creates a small, raised white bump. Because they are closed off from the air, whiteheads do not undergo oxidation and retain their white appearance.

Key Characteristics:

- Small, round, and white
- Non-inflammatory
- Typically painless

Common Areas:

- Face
- Shoulders
- Chest
- Back

Blackheads

Blackheads form when sebum and dead skin cells partially block a pore. Unlike whiteheads, the pore remains open, allowing the trapped material to undergo oxidation, which turns it black. Blackheads are often misunderstood as dirt trapped in the pores, but their dark color is due to melanin and oxidation.

Key Characteristics:

- Small, dark, and flat
- Non-inflammatory
- Can be slightly raised

Common Areas:

- Nose
- Chin
- Forehead

Papules

Papules are inflamed blemishes that appear as small, red, and tender bumps. They occur when the walls surrounding the pores break down due to severe inflammation. This leads to the formation of hard, clogged pores that are sensitive to touch.

Key Characteristics:
- Small, red, and raised
- Inflamed and tender
- No visible pus

Common Areas:
- Face
- Neck
- Shoulders
- Back

Pustules

Pustules are similar to papules but contain pus. They appear as red bumps with white or yellowish centers. Pustules form when the walls of the pores break down, leading to a build-up of white blood cells, bacteria, and dead skin cells.

Key Characteristics:
- Red with a white or yellow center
- Inflamed and tender
- Contains pus

Common Areas:

- Face
- Back
- Shoulders

Nodules

Nodules are large, painful lumps beneath the skin's surface. They form when clogged pores endure further irritation and grow larger. Nodules are hard to the touch and can be more severe than other types of acne, often requiring professional treatment.

Key Characteristics:

- Large, hard, and painful
- Deep under the skin
- No visible head

Common Areas:

- Face
- Chest
- Back

Cysts

Cysts are the most severe type of acne, characterized by large, pus-filled lesions that resemble boils. They are painful and can cause significant scarring. Cysts occur when the pores become clogged, causing a deep infection. Due to their severity, cysts often require medical intervention.

Key Characteristics:

- Large, soft, and painful
- Deep under the skin
- Filled with pus
- Can cause scarring

Common Areas:

- Face
- Neck
- Back
- Shoulders

Acne Severity

Acne can range from mild to severe, depending on the number and type of blemishes present:

- **Mild Acne:** Characterized by whiteheads and blackheads, with occasional papules and pustules.
- **Moderate Acne:** Involves more frequent papules and pustules, often spreading to the back or chest.
- **Severe Acne:** Includes numerous nodules and cysts, which can be painful and lead to scarring.

Conclusion

Understanding the different types of acne is the first step toward effective treatment and management. By recognizing each type's specific characteristics and severity, you can tailor your approach to achieve clearer, healthier skin. In the following chapters, we will explore various treatments to address and manage acne, including the potential benefits of essential oils.

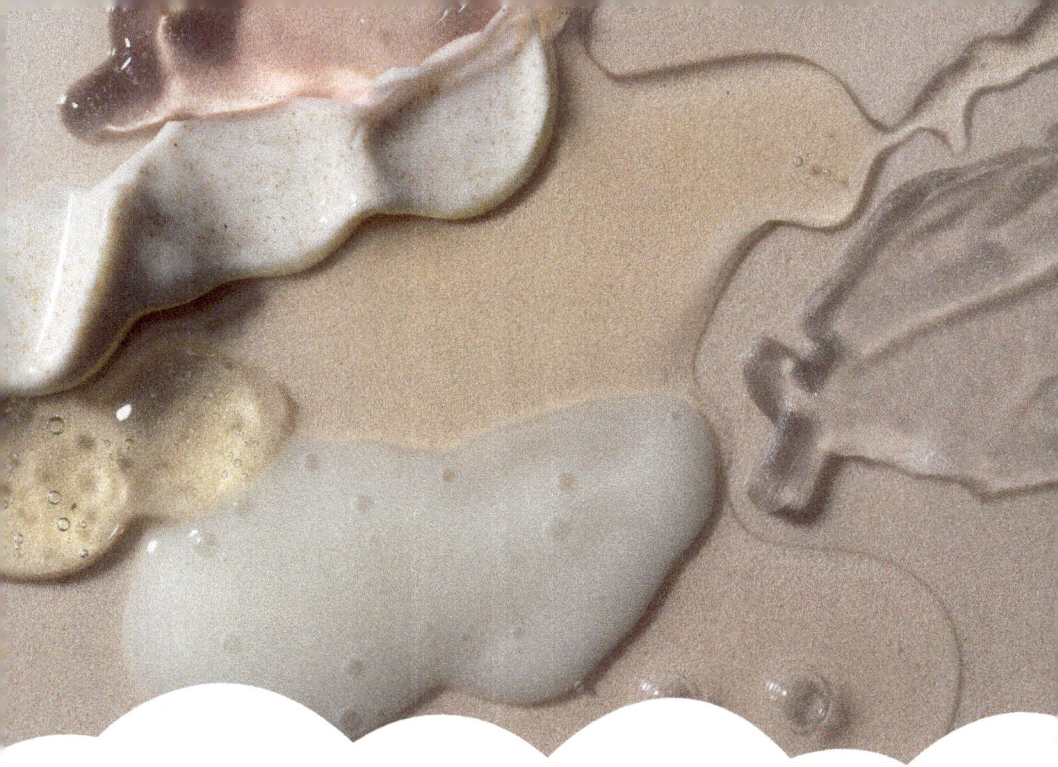

Chapter 3
Stages of Acne

Acne can be classified into different stages based on its severity and the types of lesions present. Understanding these stages can help determine the appropriate treatment and management strategies—the stages of acne range from mild to severe, each with distinct characteristics and challenges.

Mild Acne

Mild acne is the least severe form and is often the easiest to treat. It typically presents as:

- **Whiteheads:** Small, white bumps caused by sebum and dead skin cells trapped beneath the skin's surface.
- **Blackheads:** Small, dark bumps forming when sebum and dead skin cells partially block a pore and oxidize.

Mild acne may include occasional small pimples but does not involve significant inflammation.

Common Characteristics:

- Few lesions, primarily whiteheads and blackheads
- Minimal inflammation
- Typically confined to the face

Management and Treatment:

- Over-the-counter topical treatments (e.g., benzoyl peroxide, salicylic acid)
- Gentle cleansing routines
- Avoiding pore-clogging cosmetics

Moderate Acne

Moderate acne is more noticeable and may require more intensive treatment. It often includes:

- **Pimples (Papules):** Inflamed, red bumps that can be tender to the touch.
- **Pustules:** Similar to papules but contain pus, appearing as red bumps with a white or yellow center.

In moderate acne, the lesions are more widespread and can appear on the back, chest, and face.

Common Characteristics:

- More numerous lesions, including papules and pustules
- Increased inflammation
- Lesions on the face, back, and chest

Management and Treatment:

- Prescription topical treatments (e.g., retinoids, antibiotics)
- Oral medications (e.g., antibiotics, hormonal therapies)
- Consistent skincare routine

Severe Acne

Severe acne is the most intense and often the most challenging to manage. It typically includes:

- **Nodules:** Large, hard, and painful lumps beneath the skin's surface.
- **Cysts:** Large, pus-filled lesions that resemble boils and can cause significant pain and potential scarring.

Severe acne is characterized by extensive inflammation and the presence of nodules and cysts, which can cover large areas of the face, back, chest, and other body parts. This stage of acne can lead to permanent scarring if not properly treated.

Common Characteristics:

- Numerous lesions, including nodules and cysts
- Severe inflammation and pain
- Lesions on multiple areas of the body

Management and Treatment:

- Immediate consultation with a healthcare provider
- Prescription medications (e.g., oral isotretinoin)
- Potential use of corticosteroid injections for large nodules
- Professional treatments (e.g., laser therapy, chemical peels)

Gender Differences in Acne Severity

Gender plays a role in the severity and distribution of acne. Males often experience more severe acne than females due to hormonal differences, particularly the influence of androgens. Males are more prone to developing nodules and cysts, especially on the chest and back, which are typically more challenging to treat.

Key Points:

- Males are more likely to develop severe acne.
- Acne in males often appears on the chest and back.
- Hormonal fluctuations in females can also lead to significant acne, especially around the menstrual cycle.

Seeking Professional Help

For those experiencing severe or nodular acne, seeking advice from a healthcare provider is crucial. Early intervention can prevent scarring and manage the condition more effectively. Dermatologists can provide personalized treatment plans tailored to the severity of the acne and the patient's needs.

Conclusion

Understanding the stages of acne is essential for effective treatment and management. By recognizing the severity of acne and its impact on different individuals, appropriate steps can be taken to address and alleviate this common skin condition. In the following chapters, we will explore various treatments, including the potential benefits of essential oils, to help manage acne at every stage.

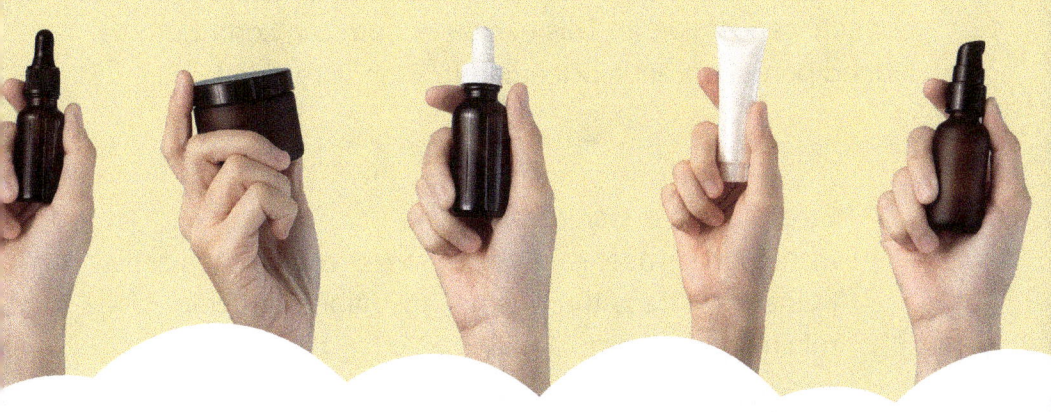

Chapter 4
Acne Myths and Truths

Many myths surround acne, leading to misconceptions about its causes and treatments. Understanding the truth behind these myths can help in managing acne more effectively. This chapter will explore some of the most common beliefs about acne and separate fact from fiction.

Myth 1: Stress Causes Acne

Truth: Stress does not directly cause acne but can exacerbate existing conditions. When stressed, your body produces more cortisol, a hormone that can increase sebum production in your sebaceous glands. This excess sebum can contribute to clogged pores, potentially leading to acne flare-ups.

Key Points:

- Stress alone doesn't cause acne.
- Increased cortisol levels from stress can worsen acne.
- Managing stress through healthy habits can help minimize flare-ups.

Note: Some medications prescribed to manage stress can have side effects that influence acne. It's important to discuss potential side effects with your healthcare provider.

Myth 2: Eating Chocolate and Greasy Foods Causes Acne

Truth: Little scientific evidence supports the claim that chocolate or greasy foods directly cause acne. However, diet can play a role in overall skin health. Foods with a high glycemic index, such as sugary snacks and refined carbohydrates, may trigger acne in some individuals by increasing insulin levels and promoting inflammation.

Key Points:

- Chocolate and greasy foods are not primary causes of acne.
- High glycemic foods may contribute to acne in some people.
- Maintaining a balanced diet can support overall skin health.

Myth 3: Dirty Skin Causes Acne

Truth: Acne is not caused by dirt. It results from clogged pores, which can be influenced by excess sebum, dead skin cells, and bacteria. Over-washing or scrubbing your face too harshly can irritate the skin and worsen acne. A gentle cleansing routine is recommended to keep the skin clean without causing irritation.

Key Points:

- Acne is not caused by dirty skin.
- Over-washing can irritate the skin and worsen acne.
- Use gentle cleansers and avoid harsh scrubbing.

Myth 4: Sun Exposure Clears Up Acne

Truth: While sun exposure can temporarily dry out pimples and reduce inflammation, it is not a long-term solution for acne. Prolonged sun exposure can damage the skin, increase the risk of skin cancer, and lead to premature aging. Additionally, sun exposure can irritate the skin, worsen existing acne problems, and cause more clogged pores as skin cells dry up and slough off quickly.

Key Points:

- Sun exposure is not a long-term solution for acne.
- Overexposure to the sun can damage the skin and worsen acne.
- Use sunscreen and follow safe sun practices.

Myth 5: Popping Pimples Helps Them Heal Faster

Truth: Popping pimples can worsen acne and lead to scarring. When you squeeze a pimple, you risk pushing bacteria and debris deeper into the skin, causing more inflammation and potential infection. Letting pimples heal naturally or seeking professional treatment if necessary is best.

Key Points:

- Popping pimples can worsen acne and cause scarring.
- It can lead to further inflammation and infection.
- Let pimples heal naturally, or seek professional treatment.

Myth 6: Only Teenagers Get Acne

Truth: Acne is commonly associated with teenagers due to hormonal changes during puberty, but it can affect people of all ages. Adult acne is a prevalent issue, often influenced by hormonal fluctuations, stress, and lifestyle factors. Women, in particular, may experience acne related to menstrual cycles, pregnancy, and menopause.

Key Points:

- Acne can affect people of all ages.
- Hormonal fluctuations can cause adult acne.
- Lifestyle and stress also play roles in adult acne.

Myth 7: Makeup Causes Acne

Truth: Not all makeup causes acne, but certain products can contribute to clogged pores, especially if they are not non-comedogenic (formulated not to block pores). Choosing the right makeup and ensuring proper skin care, including thorough makeup removal, can prevent makeup-related breakouts.

Key Points:

- Not all makeup causes acne.
- Choose non-comedogenic products to avoid clogged pores.
- Remove makeup thoroughly to prevent breakouts.

Myth 8: Acne Is Contagious

Truth: Acne is not contagious. It is a non-communicable condition, meaning no one can "catch" acne from another person. The bacteria involved in acne, *Propionibacterium acnes*, reside on everyone's skin and do not spread from person to person.

Key Points:

- Acne is not contagious.
- You cannot "catch" acne from someone else.
- Acne is a non-communicable condition.

Myth 9: You'll Outgrow Acne, So Leave It Alone

Truth: While many people experience acne during adolescence, it can affect individuals of all ages. Leaving acne untreated can lead to worsening of the condition and potential scarring. Acne is treatable at any age, and addressing it early can prevent long-term skin issues.

Key Points:

- Acne can affect people at any age.
- Untreated acne can worsen and cause scarring.
- Seek treatment to manage and prevent acne.

Myth 10: Sweating Helps Clean Out Hair Follicle Areas

Truth: Sweating does not help clean out hair follicles. In reality, strenuous activity can temporarily increase your body's oil production, worsening acne problem areas and causing recurrence or intensification of breakouts.

Key Points:

- Sweating does not clean out hair follicles.
- Increased oil production from sweating can worsen acne.
- Maintain a proper skincare routine post-exercise to manage acne.

Myth 11: Acne Problems Are Directly Proportionate to Sexual Activity

Truth: Acne is not related to sexual activity. While hormonal changes during puberty can contribute to acne, this is unrelated to sexual activity. Both adult acne and teenage acne are influenced by factors like hormones, stress, and skincare, but not by sexual activity.

Key Points:

- Acne is not related to sexual activity.
- Hormonal changes influence acne, not sexual activity.
- Focus on proper skincare and treatment for acne management.

Myth 12: People with Acne Are Dirty and Don't Wash Enough

Truth: Acne results from a buildup of oil, dead skin cells, and bacteria in a closed pore. It is not caused by dirt or lack of cleanliness. Overwashing can irritate the skin and worsen acne.

Key Points:

- Acne is not caused by dirt or lack of washing.
- Over-washing can worsen acne.
- Maintain a gentle cleansing routine.

Myth 13: Acne Is Only a Surface Issue

Truth: While acne primarily affects the skin, its impact can run deeper. Many individuals with acne experience negative social feedback, depression, and low self-esteem, which can be emotionally harmful both short-term and long-term. Acne requires proper treatment and support to address physical and emotional aspects.

Key Points:

- Acne impacts more than just the skin.
- Emotional effects can be significant and long-lasting.
- Proper treatment and support are essential.

Myth 14: There Is a Cure for Acne

Truth: There is no cure for acne, but many effective treatments are available. Prevention and management through skincare and treatment options can significantly reduce the impact of acne. Exploring the various options and finding what works best for you is important.

Key Points:

- No cure for acne exists, but treatments are effective.
- Prevention and management are essential.
- Explore available treatment options.

Myth 15: Certain Cosmetics or Spot Treatments Will Help Acne

Truth: When a blemish appears, it develops for a couple of weeks. While specific treatments can help manage acne, expecting instant results from spot treatments is unrealistic. A consistent skincare routine is more effective in the long term.

Key Points:

- Blemishes develop over weeks, not instantly.
- Spot treatments can help, but consistent skin care is vital.
- Manage expectations for acne treatments.

Myth 16: People with Acne Should Not Use Moisturizers or Makeup

Truth: Many non-comedogenic moisturizers and makeup products are specifically formulated not to clog pores. Using the right products can help maintain skin health without worsening acne. It is important to choose products designed for acne-prone skin.

Key Points:

- Non-comedogenic products are safe for acne-prone skin.
- Moisturizers and makeup can be used if chosen carefully.
- Select products designed for acne-prone skin.

Conclusion

Understanding the myths and truths about acne is crucial for effective management and treatment. You can make informed decisions about your skincare routine and treatment options by dispelling common misconceptions. In the following chapters, we will delve deeper into effective treatments and explore how essential oils can play a role in managing acne.

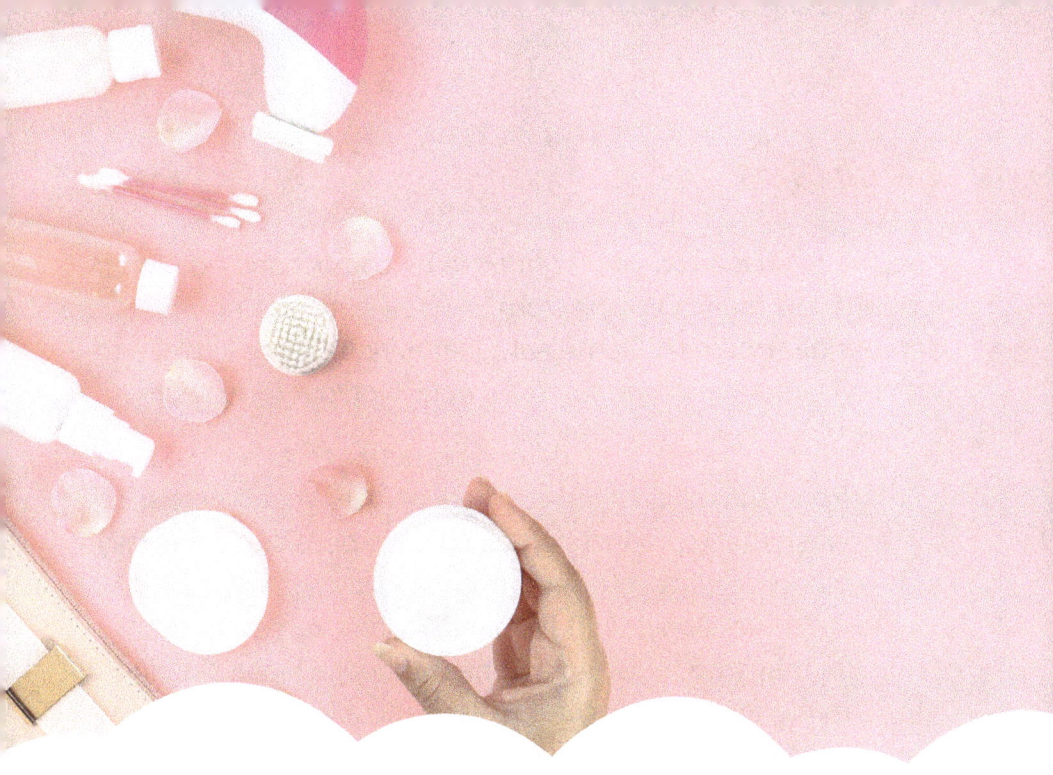

Chapter 5
Skin Care and Acne Prevention

Let's take a look at how to combat acne. The primary strategy to use is prevention where possible and better skincare. Here are several top focus issues for each: exercise, cosmetics, diet, hormones, hygiene, medications, shaving, and stress.

Exercise

Keeping in shape can help fight acne by combating negative stress levels that can come from low self-esteem and depression. However, some safeguards need to be in place to ward off acne that can result from your workout routines:

- **Watch Products:** Use "non-comedogenic" and "oil-free" sunscreens and cosmetics. After your workout, wash these products off as soon as possible, especially before using a steam room or sauna.
- **Clothing:** Avoid tight lycra and nylon exercise outfits as they trap moisture and heat. Choose loose clothing made of cotton or natural blends to allow more air to your skin. After your workout, shower and change into dry, clean clothing.
- **Gear:** Keep sports gear and equipment clean. For example, wash headbands after workout sessions.
- **Washing:** Use natural handmade soap with essential oils. When drying with a towel, blot instead of rub to avoid skin irritation.

Cosmetics

To avoid pore-clogging and skin irritations:

- Use products labeled "non-comedogenic" or "oil-free."
- Avoid shimmering facial colors containing mica, coal tar derivatives, carmine, and heavy cream.
- Use matte finish lip gloss instead of high gloss.
- Be cautious with eye creams as they can clog pores.

- Avoid hair styling products with oils, alcohol, and adhesives, especially during workouts.
- Opt for "hypo-allergenic" or "fragrance-free" cosmetics to avoid allergic reactions.

Diet

Studies show that diet does not directly cause or treat acne, but a healthy diet benefits your skin. Recommended vitamins and minerals include:

- Vitamin A: Found in liver, fish oils, dairy products, and yellowish-orange fruits and vegetables like yams and carrots.
- Vitamin B Complex: Found in leafy vegetables, fish, milk, eggs, and whole grains. B-3 (in avocados, eggs, peanuts, lean meat, and liver) helps reduce cholesterol and has anti-inflammatory effects.
- Vitamin C: Known for its antioxidant and anti-inflammatory properties.
- Vitamin E: Found in almonds, broccoli, peanuts, sunflower seeds, wheat germ, and vegetable oils.
- L-Carnitine: Helps repair skin damage from acne.
- Zinc: Found in eggs, mushrooms, nuts, and whole grains.
- Selenium: A trace mineral absorbed by various vegetables.

A good quality multivitamin combined with plenty of fluids and healthy food choices can help with acne prevention.

Hormones

Hormonal changes can play a role in acne flare-ups. Treatment options include topical retinoids, oral antibiotics, benzoyl peroxide, oral contraceptives, hormonal birth control pills, and hormone replacement therapy (HRT) for women. Consult with healthcare providers for the best options.

Hygiene

A healthy skin regimen should include:

- Avoid harsh scrubbing and over-washing.
- Use gentle exfoliation ingredients.
- Avoid alcohol-based products.
- Do not pick or squeeze blemishes.

Products

Popular products to help with acne prevention include:

- **Benzoyl Peroxide:** Destroys acne-causing bacteria.
- **Proactiv® Solution:** A 3-step acne management system.
- **Salicylic Acid:** Unclogs pores and renews skin.
- **Retinoids:** Synthetic derivatives of Vitamin A that unclog pores.
- **Antibiotics:** Destroy bacteria and decrease inflammation.
- **Oral Contraceptives:** Manage hormone levels.
- **Anti-Androgens:** Reduce sebum production.

- **Isotretinoin (Accutane):** Effective for severe cystic or nodular acne.

Shaving

Shaving can help exfoliate and remove dead skin, preventing clogged pores. For best results:

- Use shaving cream for sensitive skin.
- Moisten hair with warm water, apply shaving cream, and shave with a sharp blade.
- Use gentle swipes and shave with the grain.
- Experiment with different razors.
- Shave in a warm shower for better results.
- After shaving, use antibiotic gel, witch hazel, or other non-alcoholic toners.

Stress

Stress can affect skin health. Here's how to handle stressors:

- **External Stressors:** Avoid exposure to grease, oils, and excessive sun. Wear protective clothing and use oil-free sunscreens.
- **Internal Stressors:** Manage anxiety, fear, low self-esteem, and depression. Get plenty of rest, maintain regular hours, and reduce stress, worry, anxiety, and tension (SWAT). Keep a checklist of calming activities like reading, resting, listening to music, and taking walks.

In conclusion, a comprehensive approach that includes proper exercise, careful use of cosmetics, a healthy diet, hormone management, good hygiene, effective acne products, mindful shaving, and stress management can help prevent and combat acne.

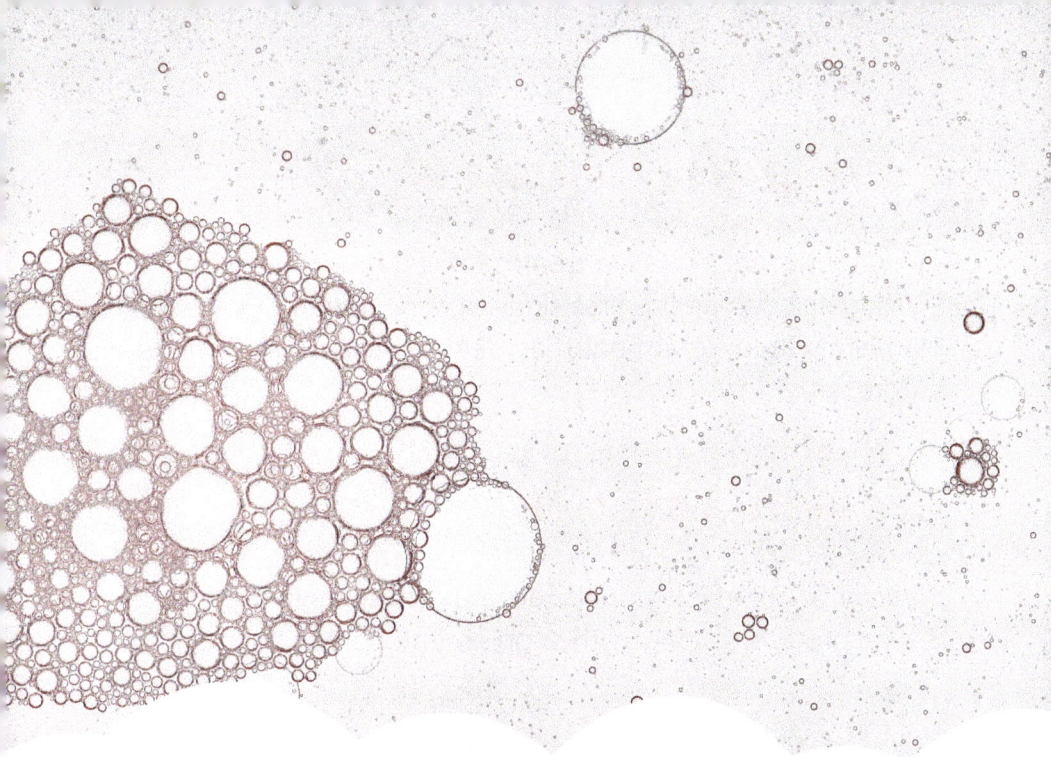

Chapter 6
Treatment with Essential Oils

There is hope. Although acne is not curable, it is treatable, and dermatologists now know more about controlling and preventing acne. One key to acne management is preventing the condition before it starts or recurs. Another is to use treatments that work best for you under the guidance of your healthcare provider or dermatologist. Natural alternative treatments with essential oils are also an option. Having covered preventative measures, let's now explore essential oil treatments.

Timing and Approach

The effectiveness of acne treatment can be enhanced by starting as soon as the first signs of acne appear. Even after blemishes fade, treatment may be necessary to prevent new outbreaks.

Proactiv Solution

Proactiv Solution is a popular acne treatment system with a 3-step program, along with supplemental products:

1. **Renewing Cleanser:** An oil-free formula containing small, smooth grains that exfoliate dead skin cells and impurities. It features prescription-grade benzoyl peroxide to penetrate pores, destroy bacteria, and heal blemishes.
2. **Revitalizing Toner:** An alcohol-free liquid with botanical agents that removes dead skin cells, balances skin tone, unplugs pores, helps control excess oil, and soothes the skin.
3. **Repairing Lotion:** A light, oil-free lotion with fine-milled prescription-grade benzoyl peroxide. It heals blackheads and blemishes and prevents future flare-ups. Its advanced delivery system is soothing and safe for the entire face.

Essential Oil Acne Treatment System

A similar approach can be taken with essential oils, which offer various healing benefits for acne. Here's an essential oil-based skincare plan modeled after the Proactiv Solution system.

This essential oil acne treatment system is a 3-step program designed to cleanse, tone, and repair acne-prone skin using natural ingredients. This plan is supplemented with additional products to support overall skin health and balance.

1. Renewing Cleanser

An all-natural exfoliating cleanser that uses the gentle power of essential oils to remove impurities, dead skin cells, and excess oil without stripping the skin of its natural moisture.

What You Will Need:

- 1/4 cup Castile soap
- 1/4 cup Distilled water
- 10 drops Tea Tree essential oil (known for its antibacterial properties)
- 5 drops Lavender essential oil (to soothe inflammation)
- 1 tablespoon Jojoba oil (balances skin's natural oils)
- 1 teaspoon fine sugar or ground oats (optional for gentle exfoliation)

Usage:

Apply a small amount to damp skin, gently massaging in circular motions to exfoliate. Rinse thoroughly with lukewarm water. Use morning and night.

2. Revitalizing Toner

An alcohol-free toner that uses botanical extracts and essential oils to balance skin tone, reduce excess oil, and tighten pores, leaving the skin feeling refreshed and revitalized.

What You Will Need:

- 1/2 cup Witch Hazel (natural astringent)
- 1/2 cup Distilled water
- 5 drops Geranium essential oil (balances oil production)
- 5 drops Lavender essential oil (calms and soothes)
- 3 drops Lemon essential oil (brightens skin and reduces excess oil)

Usage:

Apply with a cotton pad to freshly cleansed skin, avoiding the eye area. Use morning and night after cleansing.

3. Repairing Serum

A lightweight, oil-free serum that penetrates the skin deeply to repair and heal blemishes. Essential oils with antibacterial and anti-inflammatory properties help prevent future breakouts.

What You Will Need:

- 2 tablespoons Aloe Vera gel (soothes and heals)
- 1 tablespoon Rosehip Seed oil (rich in vitamins and helps repair skin)
- 10 drops Tea Tree essential oil (antibacterial)
- 5 drops Frankincense essential oil (heals and reduces scarring)

Usage:

Apply a few drops to the face, focusing on blemish-prone areas. Gently massage into the skin until fully absorbed. Use morning and night.

Supplemental Products

Oil-Free Moisturizer with SPF 15: A lightweight, non-greasy moisturizer that hydrates and protects acne-prone skin with SPF 15.

What You Will Need:

- 2 tablespoons Aloe Vera gel
- 1 tablespoon Jojoba oil (light, non-comedogenic)
- 5 drops Lavender essential oil
- 3 drops Carrot Seed essential oil (natural SPF)

Usage:

Apply a small amount to the face after the serum has been absorbed. Use in the morning as the final step in your skincare routine.

Daily Oil Control Mist: A refreshing mist that controls excess oil throughout the day, keeping skin matte and preventing makeup from smudging.

What You Will Need:

- 1/2 cup Distilled water
- 1/4 cup Witch Hazel

- 5 drops Tea Tree essential oil
- 5 drops Peppermint essential oil (refreshes and cools the skin)

Usage:

Spray lightly over the face as needed throughout the day. It can be used under or over makeup.

This essential oil-based system harnesses the natural healing power of plants to treat acne effectively and safely without the harsh chemicals found in many commercial products. Regular use can help achieve clearer, healthier skin.

Many of the recipes in this book can work well as part of an essential oil-based acne treatment system similar to the Proactiv Solution. Here's how they can be integrated into the system:

1. Cleanser:

- **Gentle Tea Tree Cleanser:** This recipe can be used as the renewing cleanser in the system. It's gentle on the skin, with Tea Tree oil providing antibacterial properties and Lavender oil offering soothing effects.

2. Toner:

- **Clarifying Lemon Toner:** This toner can replace the Revitalizing Toner. Lemon oil helps to brighten and control oil, while Eucalyptus oil helps to purify and cleanse the skin.

3. Repairing Serum:

- **Balancing Acne Serum:** The Balancing Acne Serum with Clary Sage, Tea Tree, and Rosehip Seed oil is perfect for repairing serum. It helps to balance oil production and heal blemishes.

4. Moisturizer:

- **Hydrating Acne Serum:** Although designed as a serum, it can also be used as a light moisturizer, especially if the skin needs extra hydration. Argan oil is non-comedogenic and beneficial for acne-prone skin.

5. Supplemental Products:

- **Oil-Free Moisturizer with SPF 15:** The **unscented lotion recipe** could be used as a base to create this product by adding Aloe Vera, Jojoba oil, and Carrot Seed oil for a natural SPF.

Additional Options:

- **Acne Patches:** For targeted treatment, the **acne patch** recipes provide focused care for individual blemishes, complementing the system.
- **Overnight Masks:** Overnight masks can serve as intensive treatments to calm and repair the skin during sleep.

These recipes create a comprehensive system that addresses various aspects of acne care, from cleansing and toning to repairing, moisturizing, and targeted treatments. Integrating them into a structured program can provide an effective, natural alternative to commercial acne treatment systems.

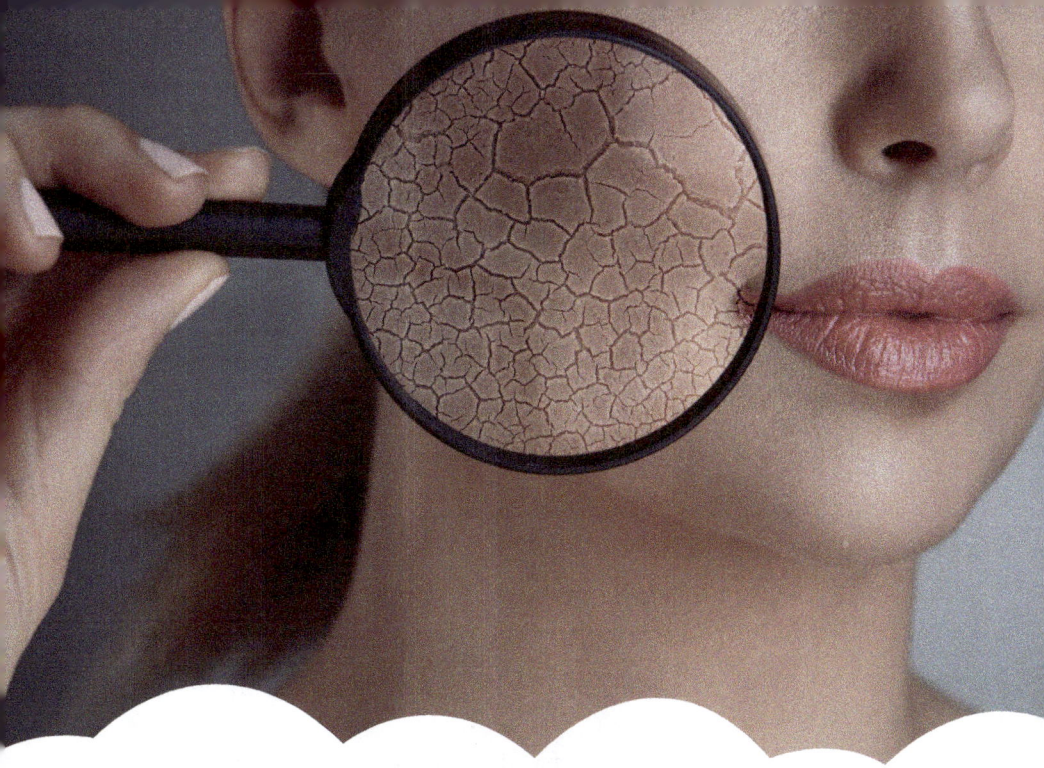

Chapter 7
Essential Oils for Skin Rejuvenation

The skin, the body's largest organ, envelops and protects the body, serving as a barrier against microorganisms and playing a crucial role in overall appearance. Despite its thin structure, the anatomy of the skin is intricate, consisting of multiple layers and various appendages, including sweat glands, hair follicles, and sebaceous (oil) glands. Essential oils, which are absorbed quickly through the skin, offer a range of benefits due to their diverse properties.

Skin Regeneration and Youthfulness

Essential oils can promote skin regeneration, contributing to a more youthful appearance. Oils known for their regenerative properties include:

- **Lavender:** Renowned for its soothing and healing effects, Lavender oil supports skin repair and rejuvenation.
- **Neroli:** Promotes cell regeneration and elasticity, making it helpful in improving the appearance of aging skin.
- **Palmarosa:** Helps balance moisture and regenerate skin cells.
- **Rosewood:** Known for its ability to stimulate the skin's natural regeneration processes.
- **Patchouli:** Enhances the healing of scars and stimulates the growth of new skin cells.

Improving Muscle Tone and Blood Circulation

Certain essential oils can enhance muscle tone and improve blood circulation, which helps prevent conditions such as varicose veins and promotes overall skin health:

- **Rosemary:** Stimulates circulation and helps tone muscles.
- **Ginger:** Known for its warming properties that stimulate blood flow.
- **Black Pepper:** Enhances circulation and improves muscle tone.

Supporting the Skin's Protective Barrier

Essential oils with acidic properties can contribute to the skin's protective barrier, helping to maintain its integrity:

- **Tea Tree:** Its slightly acidic nature supports the skin's natural defenses against pathogens.
- **Lemon:** Acts as a mild astringent, helping to tighten and tone the skin.

Anti-Inflammatory Properties

Essential oils with anti-inflammatory properties can provide relief from swelling, pain, and inflammation:

- **Lavender:** Calms inflammation and soothes irritated skin.
- **Melissa (Lemon Balm):** Reduces redness and inflammation.
- **Neroli:** Offers gentle anti-inflammatory benefits to reduce swelling and discomfort.

Balancing Sebum Production

Essential oils can help regulate sebum production, which is crucial in preventing both excessive oiliness and dryness:

- **Clary Sage:** Balances sebum production and has astringent properties.
- **Tea Tree:** Regulates sebum production and helps prevent clogged pores.

Incorporating Essential Oils into Skincare Products

Essential oils can be incorporated into various vehicles for effective delivery to the skin, including:

- **Base Creams:** Incorporating essential oils into a moisturizing base cream can provide consistent benefits for everyday use.
- **Lotions:** Light and easily absorbed, lotions with essential oils can offer hydration and treatment.
- **Gels:** Ideal for a non-greasy application, especially for oily or acne-prone skin.
- **Perfumes:** Essential oils in perfumes can offer benefits while providing a pleasant fragrance.

Recommended Essential Oils for Acne

- **Tea Tree:** Highly popular for its antimicrobial and anti-inflammatory properties, effective in treating acne, boils, and blemishes.
- **Chamomile:** Soothes the skin and reduces inflammation, ideal for calming irritated acne-prone skin.
- **Lavender:** Offers anti-inflammatory and healing properties, which are beneficial for reducing redness and promoting healing.
- **Frankincense:** Known for its skin-rejuvenating properties and ability to reduce the appearance of scars.
- **Myrrh:** Provides anti-inflammatory benefits and supports skin healing.

Essential Oils for Skin Infection and Deodorization

- **Antiseptics:** Chamomile, Lavender, Lemon, Pine, Thyme, Eucalyptus, Tea Tree, and Clove Bud effectively combat skin infections.
- **Natural Deodorants:** Bergamot, Cypress, Pine, Tea Tree, Thyme, Peppermint, Lemongrass, and Citronella can help neutralize odors and maintain skin freshness.

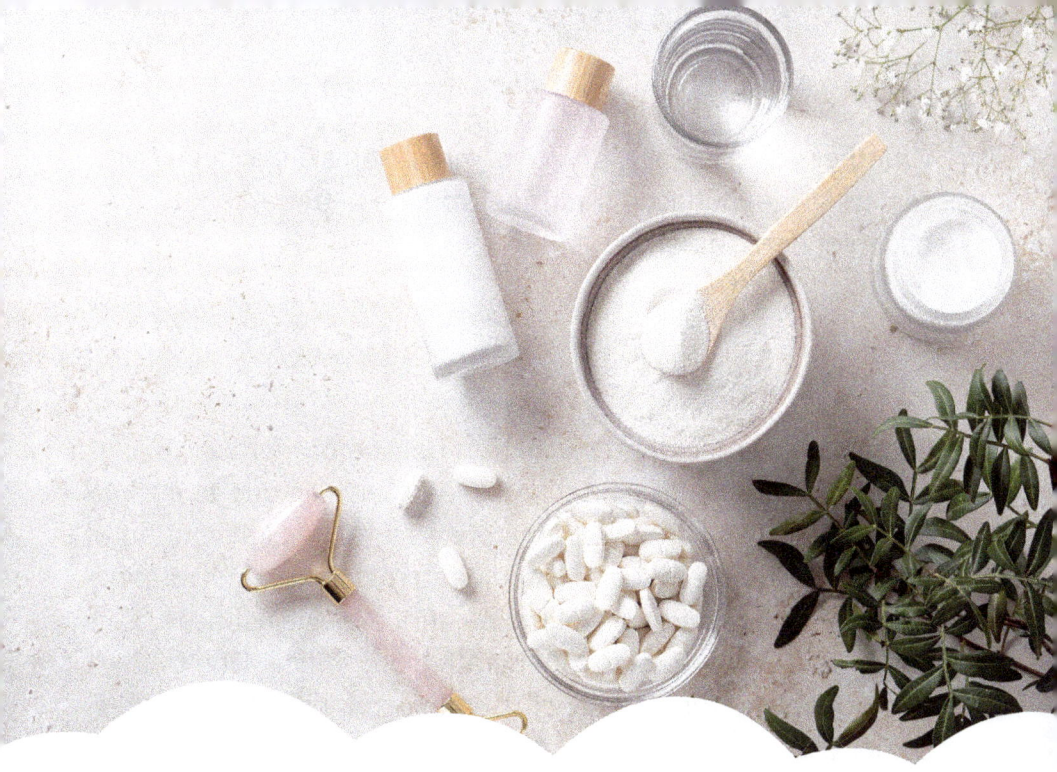

Chapter 8
Carrier Oils

Carrier oils are the foundation of many skincare products, particularly for those dealing with acne. These oils, derived from nuts, seeds, and plants, help dilute essential oils and allow for their safe application on the skin. Carrier oils offer many therapeutic benefits beyond their role as a medium for essential oils. For acne-prone skin, the right carrier oil can help balance sebum production, soothe inflammation, and support the skin's natural healing process. In this chapter, we'll explore various carrier oils that are particularly beneficial for acne, offering nourishment and protection without clogging pores.

Whether you have oily, dry, or combination skin, a carrier oil can enhance your acne treatment routine and make your skin healthier and clearer.

Tamanu Oil

Tamanu oil is renowned for its skin-healing properties and is particularly beneficial for acne-prone skin due to its antimicrobial and anti-inflammatory effects. Its high content of phospholipids and glycolipids helps to maintain skin hydration and promote repair. This oil is also effective against acne scars and blemishes due to its regenerative properties. Due to its thick, grainy texture, it is best used in combination with other carrier oils.

- **Dilution:** Use 10-50% dilution for acne treatment with another carrier oil or carrier oil blend. Tamanu oil can be blended with lighter oils like Jojoba or Grapeseed for easier application.

Jojoba Oil

Jojoba oil closely resembles the skin's natural sebum, making it effective for balancing oil production and preventing clogged pores. Its anti-inflammatory properties are beneficial for reducing acne-related redness and swelling. Jojoba oil is also known for dissolving excess sebum, making it a good choice for oily and acne-prone skin. It helps to cleanse the skin and promote a clear complexion.

- **Dilution:** It can be used at 100%, but due to its cost, it is common practice to use a 10% dilution with other carrier oils.

Grapeseed Oil

Grapeseed oil is a light, non-greasy oil ideal for acne-prone skin due to its astringent properties, which help tighten and tone the skin. Its natural anti-inflammatory and antioxidant properties effectively reduce acne inflammation and prevent breakouts. Grapeseed oil also helps to balance oil production without leaving a greasy residue.

- **Dilution:** This can be used at 100%, but mixing with other oils can enhance its benefits for acne-prone skin.

Argan Oil

Argan oil is rich in essential fatty acids and Vitamin E, which provide excellent hydration without clogging pores. It helps to reduce inflammation and soothe irritated skin, making it beneficial for acne and related skin conditions. Argan oil's ability to balance sebum production makes it effective for dry and oily acne-prone skin. It can also be combined with Pomegranate Seed oil for enhanced antioxidant protection.

- **Dilution:** Can be used at 100% or blended with other oils for a customized acne treatment.

Rosehip Seed Oil

Rosehip Seed oil is rich in essential fatty acids and Vitamin A, effectively reducing acne scars and promoting skin regeneration. It helps to balance oil production and improve skin texture, making it a good choice for acne-prone skin.

- Dilution: Typically used at 10-20% in a carrier oil blend.

Calendula Oil

Calendula oil has strong anti-inflammatory and antimicrobial properties, making it excellent for soothing irritated acne-prone skin and reducing redness. It also aids in the healing of acne scars.

- Dilution: Can be used at 10-30% in a carrier oil blend.

Hemp Seed Oil

Hemp Seed oil balances the skin's oil production and reduces acne. It is rich in essential fatty acids and has anti-inflammatory properties that help to calm the skin and reduce breakouts.

- Dilution: Can be used at 100% or mixed with other oils.

These carrier oils can be combined with essential oils for targeted acne treatment and to address specific skin concerns.

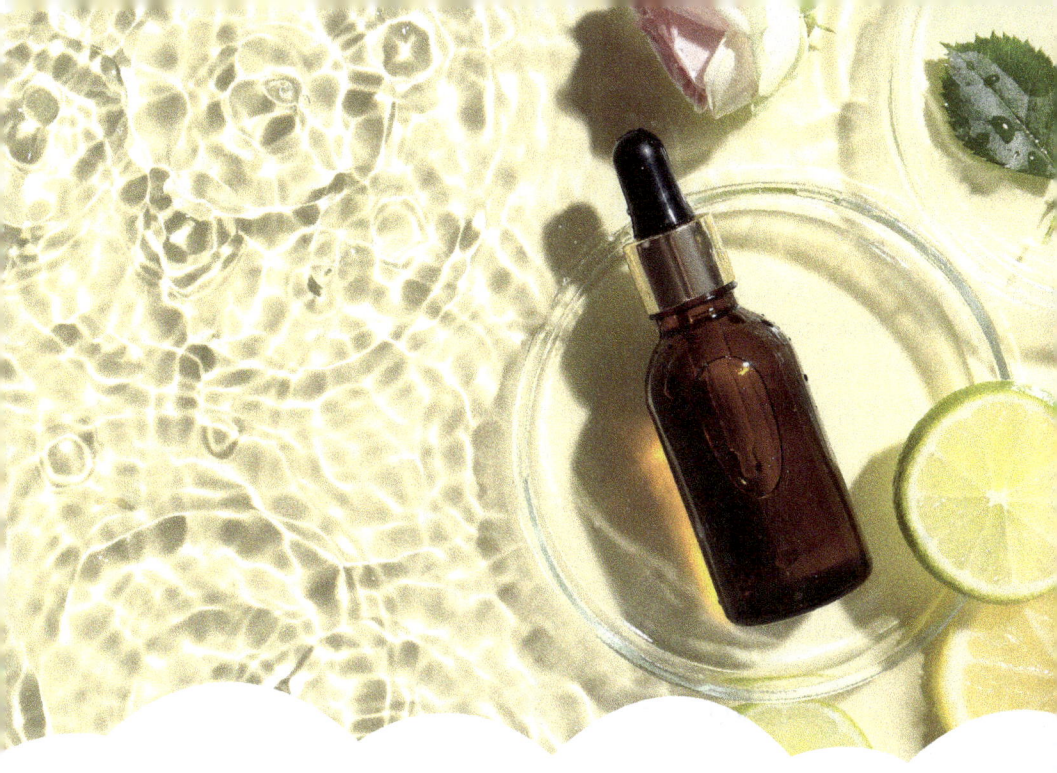

Chapter 9
Essential Oils for Acne

Acne can be a persistent and frustrating challenge, but the right treatments can make a significant difference in managing and improving the condition of your skin. Essential oils offer a powerful alternative to conventional acne treatments with their natural healing properties. They have been celebrated not only for their ability to address the symptoms of acne but also for their broader benefits in skin care.

In this book, we will explore a variety of recipes that utilize essential oils and natural ingredients to tackle acne. Each recipe has been carefully crafted to address different aspects of acne management, from reducing inflammation and combating bacteria to soothing irritated skin and promoting healing.

You will find a range of treatments, including facial scrubs, masks, and serums, all designed to integrate the therapeutic benefits of essential oils into your skincare routine. Whether you're looking for a gentle daily cleanser or a deep-cleansing mask, these recipes will guide you in creating effective and natural skincare solutions.

By incorporating these recipes into your routine, you can harness the power of essential oils to improve your skin's health and appearance. Let's delve into these essential oils and discover how to create effective, natural remedies for acne.

Acne

Essential oils in this chart are known for their ability to soothe inflammation, balance sebum production, and promote clear, healthy skin, making them effective for treating various types of acne.

Top	Middle	Base
Basil	Chamomile, Roman	Benzoin
Bergamot	Chamomile, German	Cedarwood
Cajeput	Clove Bud	Frankincense
Camphor	Carrot Seed	Helichrysum

Clary Sage	Cypress	Jasmine
Eucalyptus	Geranium	Myrrh
Galbanum	Juniper Berry	Patchouli
Grapefruit	Lavender	Rose
Lemon	Linaloe Berry	Rosewood
Lemongrass	Melissa	Sandalwood
Lime	Myrtle	Spikenard
May Chang	Neroli	Tarragon
Mandarin	Niaouli	Vetiver
Peppermint	Palmarosa	Violet
Petitgrain	Rosemary	Ylang Ylang
Orange	Rose Geranium	
Sage	Spruce	
Spearmint	Thyme	
Tea Tree	Yarrow	

Astringent

Acne is one of the most common skin problems worldwide. Astringents used topically shrink or tighten pores, preventing toxins and dirt from getting in. They are also used to remove oil from the skin easily.

Top	Middle	Base
Bay Laurel	Bay	Benzoin
Birch	Caraway Seed	Cedarwood
Cedar Leaf	Cinnamon	Frankincense
Citronella	Cypress	Myrrh

Clary Sage	Geranium	Opoponax
Fleabane	Hyssop	Patchouli
Grapefruit	Juniper Berry	Rose
Lemon	Lavender	Sandalwood
Lemongrass	Myrtle	
Lime	Parsley	
Peppermint	Plai	
Orange	Rosemary	
Spearmint	Rose Geranium	
Sage	Yarrow	
Tea Tree		

Blackheads and Pimples

Blackheads and pimples, common forms of acne, occur when pores become clogged with excess oil, dead skin cells, and bacteria; essential oils below can help control oil production and kill acne-causing bacteria.

Top	Middle	Base
Lemon	Cajeput	
Lemongrass	Coriander	
Niaouli	Geranium	
Peppermint	German Chamomile	
Sweet Orange	Helichrysum	
Tea Tree	Lemon Myrtle	
	Oregano (spot only)	
	Palmarosa	

	Rosemary	
	Thyme Linalool	

Scars

Essential oils in this chart are selected for their potential to promote skin regeneration and reduce the appearance of acne scars, aiding in the healing process and improving skin texture.

Top	Middle	Base
Petitgrain	Carrot Seed	Galbanum
	Helichrysum (in a base of Rosehip Seed oil)	
	Lavender	

Inflammation

Essential oils in this chart are known for their anti-inflammatory properties, helping to soothe irritated skin and reduce the redness and swelling associated with acne.

Top	Middle	Base
Myrtle (to middle)	Angelica	Cistus Labdanum
	German Chamomile	Galbanum
	Roman Chamomile	Myrrh
	Carrot Seed	Yarrow
	Clary Sage	
	Helichrysum	
	Rosewood	

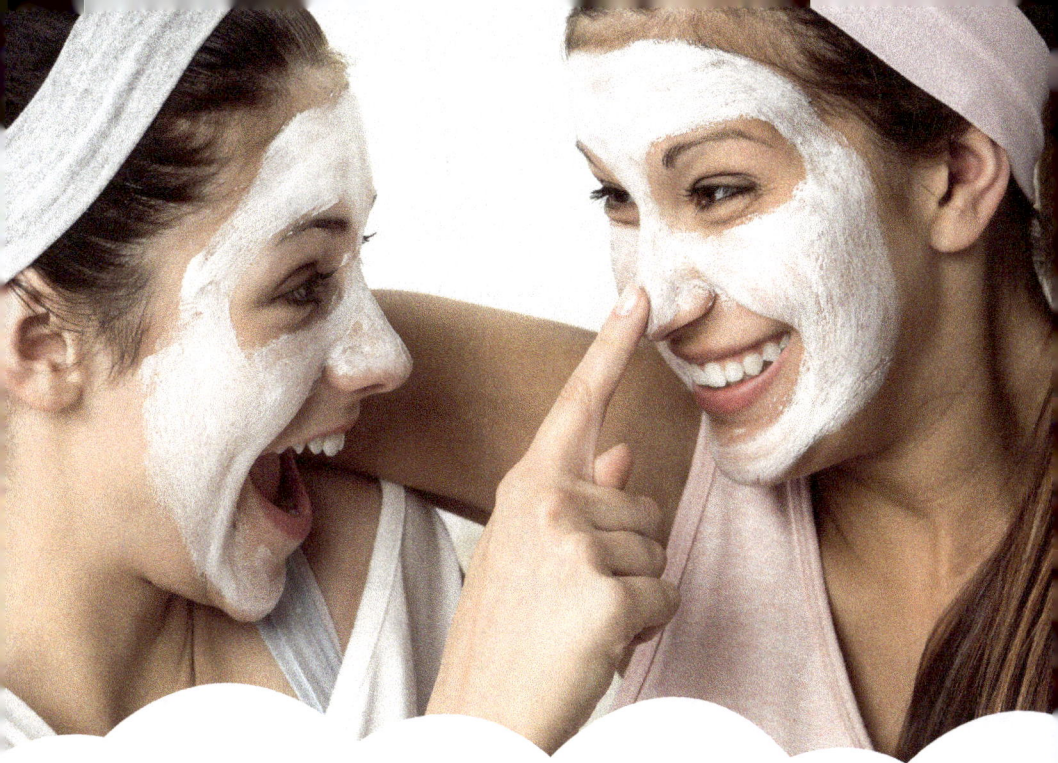

Chapter 10
Facial Masks

Facial masks offer a powerful way to address acne and enhance skin health, providing targeted treatments beyond daily cleansing. In this section, you'll discover a variety of facial mask recipes designed to combat acne using essential oils and natural ingredients. These masks work by drawing out impurities, soothing inflammation, and providing essential nutrients that help clear and heal the skin.

Each mask recipe addresses different aspects of acne care, from reducing excess oil and unclogging pores to calming redness and irritation. Whether you're dealing with occasional breakouts or persistent acne, these masks can be integrated into your skincare routine to achieve healthier skin. Prepare to pamper your skin with these natural remedies, and find the perfect mask to fit your unique needs.

Tea Tree and Honey Facial Mask

This recipe combines the antimicrobial benefits of tea tree oil with honey's soothing and hydrating properties, making it an effective treatment for reducing acne and calming inflamed skin.

What You Will Need:

- 1 tablespoon Honey
- 1 teaspoon Tea Tree oil
- 1 teaspoon Aloe Vera gel
- Small mixing bowl
- Measuring spoons
- Stirring utensil (spoon or spatula)
- Clean face brush or applicator (optional)
- Clean towel

What To Do:

1. In a small mixing bowl, combine the honey and aloe vera gel.
2. Add the tea tree oil and stir well.
3. Apply the mask evenly to your face using a clean face brush or applicator if desired.
4. Leave the mask on for 10-15 minutes, then rinse off with warm water.
5. Pat your face dry with a clean towel.

Bentonite Clay and Lemon Mask

This recipe uses the purifying power of bentonite clay to detoxify and absorb excess oil. In contrast, lemon oil provides astringent and brightening effects, making it ideal for clarifying and treating acne-prone skin.

What You Will Need:

- 2 tablespoons Bentonite Clay
- 1 tablespoon Apple Cider Vinegar
- 1 teaspoon Lemon essential oil
- Water (as needed)
- Measuring spoons
- Stirring utensil (spoon or spatula)
- Non-metallic bowl (bentonite clay reacts with metal)
- Clean towel

What To Do:

1. Combine the bentonite clay and apple cider vinegar in a non-metallic mixing bowl.
2. Add the lemon essential oil and stir.
3. Slowly add water until a smooth paste forms.
4. Apply the mask evenly to your face and let it dry for 10-15 minutes.
5. Rinse off with warm water and follow with moisturizer.

Charcoal and Eucalyptus Mask

This mask combines activated charcoal, which helps draw out impurities and unclog pores, with eucalyptus oil's soothing and antibacterial properties, making it an excellent choice for purifying and calming acne-prone skin.

What You Will Need:

- 1 tablespoon Activated Charcoal powder
- 1 tablespoon Coconut oil
- 2 drops Eucalyptus essential oil
- Small mixing bowl
- Measuring spoons
- Stirring utensil (spoon or spatula)
- Clean face brush or applicator (optional)
- Clean towel

What To Do:

1. Mix the activated charcoal powder and coconut oil in a small mixing bowl.
2. Add the eucalyptus essential oil and stir until combined.
3. If desired, apply the mask to your face using a clean face brush or applicator.
4. Leave the mask on for 10 minutes, then rinse thoroughly with warm water.
5. Pat your face dry with a clean towel.

Yogurt and Peppermint Face Mask

This mask blends soothing yogurt with cooling peppermint oil to help reduce inflammation and irritation, providing a refreshing and calming treatment for acne-prone skin.

What You Will Need:

- 2 tablespoons Plain Yogurt
- 1 teaspoon Honey
- 2 drops Peppermint essential oil
- Small mixing bowl
- Measuring spoons
- Stirring utensil (spoon or spatula)
- Clean face brush or applicator (optional)
- Clean towel

What To Do:

1. In a small mixing bowl, combine the yogurt and honey.
2. Add the peppermint essential oil and stir well.
3. Apply the mixture to your face using a clean face brush or applicator if desired.
4. Leave the mask on for 10-15 minutes, then rinse with lukewarm water.
5. Pat your face dry with a clean towel.

Aloe Vera and Clove Bud Mask

This recipe combines the soothing properties of aloe vera with the antiseptic benefits of clove bud oil; this mask helps calm and treat acne while promoting skin healing.

What You Will Need:

- 2 tablespoons Aloe Vera gel
- 1 teaspoon Honey
- 2 drops Clove Bud essential oil
- Small mixing bowl
- Measuring spoons
- Stirring utensil (spoon or spatula)
- Clean face brush or applicator (optional)
- Clean towel

What To Do:

1. In a small mixing bowl, mix the aloe vera gel and honey.
2. Add the clove bud essential oil and stir well.
3. Apply the mask evenly to your face using a clean face brush or applicator if desired.
4. Leave the mask on for 10 minutes, then rinse off with lukewarm water.
5. Pat your face dry with a clean towel.

Cucumber and Chamomile Refreshing Mask

Infused with cucumber and chamomile, this mask provides a cooling, soothing effect that helps calm irritated skin and reduce inflammation from acne.

What You Will Need:

- 1/2 Cucumber (blended into a puree)
- 1 tablespoon Chamomile Tea (cooled)
- 1 tablespoon Plain Yogurt
- Blender or food processor
- Small mixing bowl
- Measuring spoons
- Stirring utensil (spoon or spatula)
- Clean face brush or applicator (optional)
- Clean towel

What To Do:

1. Blend the cucumber into a smooth puree.
2. Combine the cucumber puree, chamomile tea, and plain yogurt in a small mixing bowl.
3. Apply the mask evenly to your face using a clean face brush or applicator if desired.
4. Leave the mask on for 15 minutes, then rinse with cool water.
5. Pat your face dry with a clean towel.

Tea Tree and Bentonite Clay Mask

This mask combines bentonite clay's purifying properties with tea tree oil's antimicrobial benefits to help detoxify the skin and target acne-causing bacteria.

What You Will Need:

- 2 tablespoons Bentonite Clay
- 1 tablespoon Distilled water
- 5 drops Tea Tree oil
- 1 teaspoon Honey
- Non-metallic bowl (bentonite clay reacts with metal)
- Mixing utensil (spoon or spatula)
- Clean brush or fingers for application
- Clean towel

What To Do:

1. To form a paste, combine bentonite clay with distilled water in a small non-metallic bowl.
2. Add tea tree oil and honey and mix thoroughly.
3. Apply the mask evenly to your face using a clean brush or fingers, avoiding the eye area.
4. Leave on for 10-15 minutes before rinsing with warm water. Pat dry with a clean towel.

Neem and Turmeric Mask

This mask utilizes neem and turmeric's antibacterial and anti-inflammatory properties to combat acne and reduce redness, promoting a clearer, more balanced complexion.

What You Will Need:

- 1 tablespoon Neem powder
- 1 tablespoon Turmeric powder
- 1 tablespoon Yogurt
- 5 drops Lavender essential oil
- Small mixing bowl
- Mixing utensil (spoon or spatula)
- Clean brush or fingers for application
- Clean towel

What To Do:

1. In a small bowl, mix neem powder and turmeric powder with yogurt to create a thick paste.
2. Add lavender oil and stir well.
3. Apply the mask to your face using a clean brush or your fingers.
4. Let it sit for 10 minutes before rinsing with lukewarm water. Follow with a gentle moisturizer.

Ginger and Green Tea Mask

This mask combines ginger's anti-inflammatory benefits with green tea's antioxidant properties to soothe irritated skin and reduce acne while promoting overall skin health.

What You Will Need:

- 2 tablespoons Green Tea (brewed and cooled)
- 1 tablespoon Ginger powder
- 1 teaspoon Honey
- 5 drops Frankincense essential oil
- Small mixing bowl
- Mixing utensil (spoon or spatula)
- Clean brush or fingers for application
- Clean towel

What To Do:

1. Combine brewed and cooled green tea with ginger powder in a small bowl.
2. Add honey and frankincense oil, mixing until smooth.
3. Apply the mask to your face using a clean brush or your fingers.
4. Leave on for 15 minutes before rinsing with warm water. Pat your face dry with a clean towel.

Yogurt and Sandalwood Mask

This mask blends yogurt's hydrating and soothing properties with sandalwood's anti-inflammatory and antiseptic benefits to calm acne-prone skin and promote a clearer complexion.

What You Will Need:

- 2 tablespoons Plain Yogurt
- 1 tablespoon Sandalwood powder
- 1 teaspoon Honey
- 5 drops Clary Sage essential oil
- Small mixing bowl
- Mixing utensil (spoon or spatula)
- Clean brush or fingers for application
- Clean towel

What To Do:

1. In a small bowl, mix yogurt and sandalwood powder until well combined.
2. Stir in honey and clary sage oil.
3. Apply the mask to your face using a clean brush or your fingers, avoiding sensitive areas around the eyes.
4. Leave it on for 10-15 minutes before rinsing with lukewarm water. Pat your face dry with a clean towel.

Tea Tree and Lavender Overnight Mask

This overnight mask combines the purifying effects of tea tree oil with lavender's calming and healing properties, helping to reduce acne and promote skin rejuvenation while you sleep.

What You Will Need:

- 1 tablespoon Aloe Vera Gel
- 5 drops Tea Tree essential oil
- 5 drops Lavender essential oil
- Small mixing bowl
- Clean spatula or spoon
- Airtight container for storage

What To Do:

1. Combine aloe vera gel with tea tree and lavender oils in a small mixing bowl.
2. Mix until all ingredients are well blended.
3. Apply a thin layer to your face before bed, focusing on acne-prone areas.
4. Leave the mask on overnight and rinse off with lukewarm water in the morning.
5. Store any remaining mask in an airtight container.

Chamomile and Honey Overnight Mask

This overnight mask blends the soothing properties of chamomile with honey's moisturizing and antibacterial benefits, calming irritation and hydrating the skin while you rest.

What You Will Need:

- 1 tablespoon raw Honey
- 5 drops Roman Chamomile essential oil
- 1 teaspoon Jojoba oil
- Small mixing bowl
- Clean spatula or spoon
- Airtight container for storage

What To Do:

1. Mix raw honey, chamomile, and jojoba oils in a small bowl until smooth.
2. Apply a thin, even layer to your face, concentrating on acne-prone areas.
3. Leave the mask on overnight and rinse with warm water in the morning.
4. Store any leftover mixture in an airtight container.

Frankincense and Rose Water Overnight Mask

This overnight mask combines the rejuvenating effects of frankincense with the hydrating and soothing properties of rose water, promoting skin repair and reducing the appearance of blemishes as you sleep.

What You Will Need:

- 1 tablespoon Rose Water
- 5 drops Frankincense essential oil
- 1 teaspoon Bentonite Clay
- Non-metallic bowl
- Clean spatula or spoon
- Airtight container for storage

What To Do:

1. Mix rose water with frankincense oil and bentonite clay in a small non-metallic bowl until it forms a smooth paste.
2. Apply the mask to your face, focusing on areas with acne.
3. Allow the mask to dry slightly before bed, then leave it on overnight.
4. Rinse off with warm water in the morning.
5. Store any remaining mask in an airtight container.

Peppermint and Green Tea Overnight Mask

This overnight mask blends invigorating peppermint with soothing green tea, offering a cooling effect that calms irritated skin while reducing inflammation and promoting healing throughout the night.

What You Will Need:

- 1 tablespoon cooled brewed Green Tea
- 5 drops Peppermint essential oil
- 1 teaspoon Aloe Vera gel
- Small mixing bowl
- Clean spatula or spoon
- Airtight container for storage

What To Do:

1. Combine cooled tea, peppermint oil, and aloe vera gel in a small bowl.
2. Mix well until ingredients are thoroughly combined.
3. Apply the mask to your face before bedtime, focusing on inflamed areas.
4. Leave it on overnight and rinse off with lukewarm water in the morning.
5. Store any remaining mask in an airtight container.

Rosemary and Clay Overnight Mask

This overnight mask combines rosemary with clay to detoxify and purify the skin, helping to absorb excess oil and refine pores while delivering antibacterial and anti-inflammatory benefits as you sleep.

What You Will Need:

- 1 tablespoon Bentonite Clay
- 5 drops Rosemary essential oil
- 1 teaspoon Apple Cider Vinegar
- Water (as needed)
- Non-metallic bowl (bentonite clay reacts with metal)
- Clean spatula or spoon
- Airtight container for storage

What To Do:

1. Mix bentonite clay with rosemary oil and apple cider vinegar in a small non-metallic bowl.
2. Add water gradually to achieve a smooth, spreadable consistency.
3. Apply the mask to your face, focusing on acne-prone areas.
4. Leave the mask on overnight and rinse off with warm water in the morning.
5. Store any remaining mask in an airtight container.

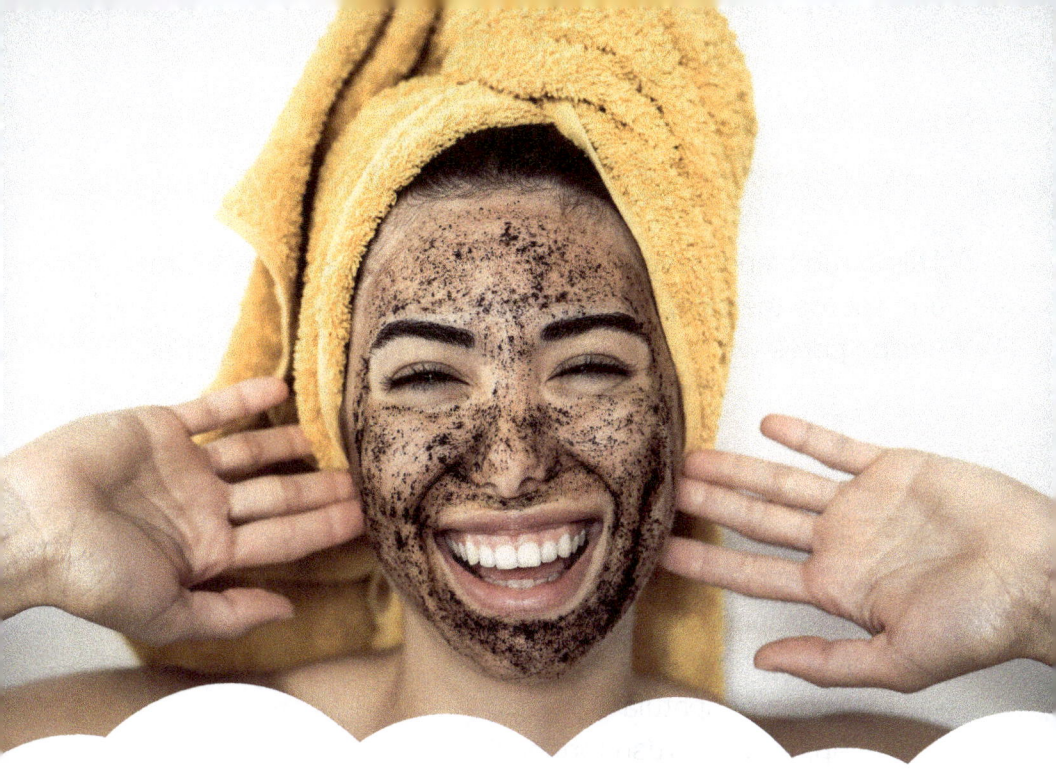

Chapter 11
Exfoliating Scrubs

Exfoliating scrubs are crucial in maintaining healthy, clear skin, especially for those dealing with acne. By gently removing dead skin cells, excess oil, and impurities from the surface, these scrubs help to unclog pores and prevent breakouts. This section explores creating exfoliating scrubs using natural ingredients and essential oils tailored to address acne concerns. You'll learn how to formulate scrubs that not only exfoliate but also soothe and treat acne-prone skin, promoting a smoother, more radiant complexion. Whether you're looking to brighten dull skin or reduce the frequency of breakouts, these homemade exfoliating scrubs offer a customized approach to achieving clearer, healthier skin.

Lavender and Oatmeal Scrub

This scrub blends lavender and oatmeal to gently exfoliate and soothe the skin, helping to reduce acne inflammation and unclog pores while providing a calming and hydrating effect.

What You Will Need:

- 2 tablespoons finely ground Oatmeal
- 1 tablespoon Honey
- 1 teaspoon Lavender essential oil
- 1 teaspoon Yogurt
- Mixing bowl
- Spoon or spatula
- Application brush (optional)
- Towel
- Jar or container with a lid (if you're preparing more than one use)

What To Do:

1. Combine the oatmeal and honey in a mixing bowl.
2. Add the lavender essential oil and yogurt and mix until smooth.
3. Gently massage the scrub onto your face in circular motions for 1-2 minutes.
4. Rinse with lukewarm water and pat dry.
5. This scrub can be stored in a clean, airtight container if not used immediately. Use it within a week if stored, and keep it in a cool, dry place.

Tea Tree and Coconut Scrub

This scrub combines tea tree oil and coconut to cleanse and exfoliate the skin, harnessing tea tree's antibacterial properties to target acne. In contrast, coconut oil provides gentle moisturizing and soothing benefits.

What You Will Need:

- 1/2 cup Coconut oil
- 1/2 cup Granulated Sugar or Sea Salt
- 10 drops Tea Tree essential oil
- 5 drops Lavender essential oil
- Mixing bowl
- Spoon or spatula
- Jar or container with a lid

What To Do:

1. Melt the coconut oil if solid.
2. Mix the melted coconut oil with the sugar or salt.
3. Add tea tree and lavender oils.
4. Stir well and transfer to a jar.
5. Gently massage onto damp skin, then rinse with warm water.

Lemon and Honey Exfoliating Mask

This mask blends lemon's natural astringent properties with honey's soothing and moisturizing effects to help exfoliate dead skin cells, brighten the complexion, and reduce the appearance of acne scars.

What You Will Need:

- 1/4 cup Honey
- 1/4 cup finely ground Oats
- 10 drops Lemon essential oil
- 5 drops Frankincense essential oil
- Mixing bowl
- Spoon
- Application brush (optional)
- Towel

What To Do:

1. Mix honey and ground oats in a bowl.
2. Add lemon and frankincense oils.
3. Stir until well combined.
4. Apply to the face, gently massaging in circular motions.
5. Leave on for 10 minutes, then rinse with warm water.

Green Tea and Matcha Scrub

This scrub combines green tea's antioxidant-rich properties with matcha's exfoliating benefits to gently polish the skin, unclog pores, and reduce inflammation, promoting a clearer and more radiant complexion.

What You Will Need:

- 1/4 cup Green Tea (cooled)
- 1/4 cup Matcha powder
- 2 tablespoons Sugar
- 5 drops Peppermint essential oil
- Mixing bowl
- Spoon
- Jar or container for storage

What To Do:

1. Combine green tea and matcha powder in a bowl.
2. Add sugar and peppermint oil.
3. Mix until a paste forms.
4. Gently apply to the face and scrub in circular motions.
5. Rinse thoroughly with lukewarm water.

Aloe Vera and Rose Scrub

This scrub blends aloe vera's soothing and hydrating properties with the gentle exfoliation of rose petals to calm irritation, remove dead skin cells, and rejuvenate the complexion, making it ideal for sensitive or acne-prone skin.

What You Will Need:

- 1/4 cup Aloe Vera gel
- 1/4 cup finely ground Almonds
- 10 drops Rose essential oil
- 5 drops Roman Chamomile essential oil
- Mixing bowl
- Spoon
- Jar or container with a lid

What To Do:

1. Combine aloe vera gel and ground almonds in a bowl.
2. Add rose and chamomile oils.
3. Stir until evenly mixed.
4. Apply to the face, gently massaging in circular motions.
5. Rinse with warm water.

Bentonite Clay and Lavender Cream

This cream combines the purifying properties of bentonite clay with the soothing effects of lavender to detoxify the skin, reduce inflammation, and promote a calm, clear complexion, making it perfect for addressing acne and balancing the skin.

What You Will Need:

- 1/4 cup Bentonite Clay
- 1/4 cup Plain Yogurt
- 10 drops Lavender essential oil
- 5 drops Tea Tree essential oil
- Non-metallic bowl (bentonite clay reacts with metal)
- Spoon
- Application brush (optional)
- Towel

What To Do:

1. Mix bentonite clay and yogurt in a non-metallic bowl until smooth.
2. Add lavender and tea tree oils.
3. Apply to the face, avoiding the eye area.
4. Leave on for 10 minutes, then rinse with warm water.

Mint and Sea Salt Scrub

This invigorating scrub blends sea salt with refreshing mint to gently exfoliate dead skin cells, unclog pores, and soothe inflammation, providing a revitalizing treatment for acne-prone skin.

What You Will Need:

- 1/2 cup Sea Salt
- 1/4 cup Olive oil
- 10 drops Peppermint essential oil
- 5 drops Eucalyptus essential oil
- Mixing bowl
- Spoon or spatula
- Jar or container with a lid

What To Do:

1. Mix sea salt and olive oil in a bowl.
2. Add peppermint and eucalyptus oils.
3. Stir until well combined.
4. Gently massage onto damp skin.
5. Rinse with warm water.

Oatmeal and Tea Tree Exfoliating Cream

This exfoliating cream combines soothing oatmeal with antibacterial tea tree oil to gently remove dead skin cells, reduce acne-causing bacteria, and calm irritated skin, making it an ideal treatment for maintaining clear, healthy skin.

What You Will Need:

- 1/2 cup finely ground Oatmeal
- 1/4 cup Shea Butter
- 10 drops Tea Tree essential oil
- 5 drops Lemon essential oil
- Mixing bowl
- Spoon or spatula
- Jar or container with a lid

What To Do:

1. Melt the shea butter if solid.
2. Mix with ground oatmeal.
3. Add tea tree and lemon oils.
4. Stir well and transfer to a jar.
5. Apply to the face, gently scrubbing in circular motions.
6. Rinse thoroughly with lukewarm water.

Honey and Lemon Sugar Scrub

This invigorating sugar scrub blends honey and lemon to exfoliate dead skin cells, brighten the complexion, and balance oil production, helping to reduce acne and leave the skin smooth and refreshed.

What You Will Need:

- 1/4 cup Honey
- 1/4 cup Granulated Sugar
- 10 drops Lemon essential oil
- 5 drops Lavender essential oil
- Mixing bowl
- Spoon
- Jar or container with a lid

What To Do:

1. Mix honey and sugar in a bowl.
2. Add lemon and lavender oils.
3. Stir until well combined.
4. Gently massage onto damp skin.
5. Rinse with warm water.

Coconut and Activated Charcoal Scrub

This detoxifying scrub combines coconut oil and activated charcoal to deeply cleanse pores, draw out impurities, and gently exfoliate, making it ideal for acne-prone skin.

What You Will Need:

- 1/2 cup Coconut oil
- 1/4 cup Granulated Sugar
- 1 tablespoon Activated Charcoal powder
- 10 drops Tea Tree essential oil
- Mixing bowl
- Spoon or spatula
- Jar or container with a lid

What To Do:

1. Melt the coconut oil if solid.
2. Mix with sugar and activated charcoal powder.
3. Add tea tree oil.
4. Stir until well combined.
5. Apply to the face, gently scrubbing in circular motions.
6. Rinse with warm water.

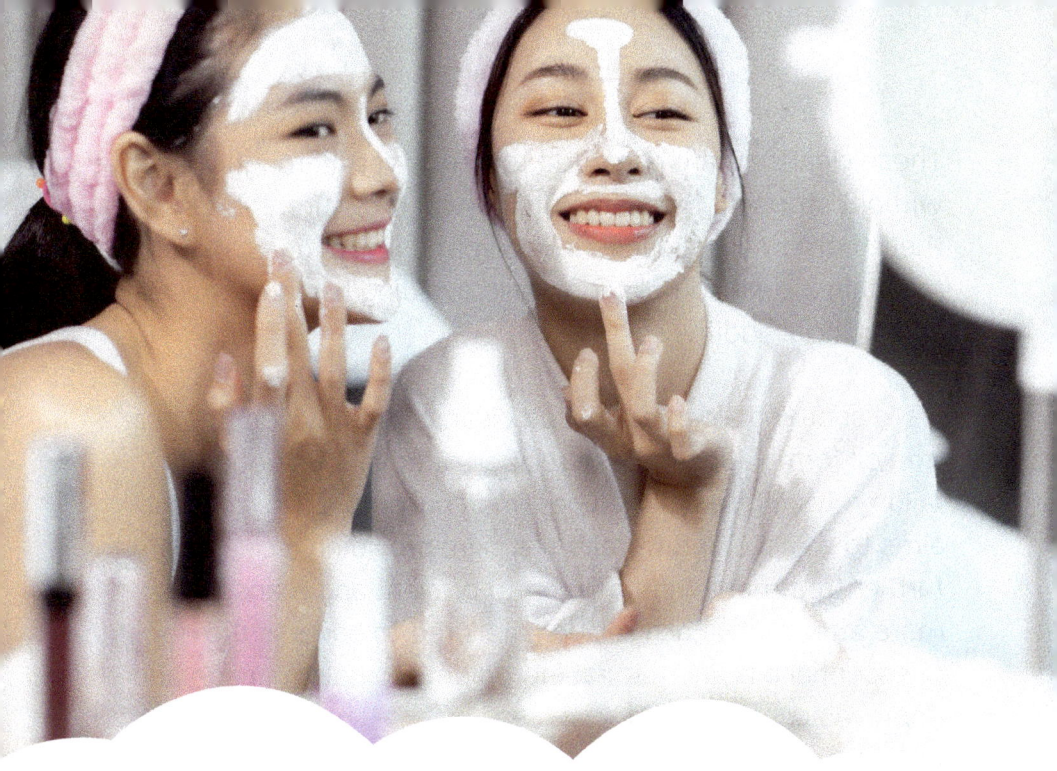

Chapter 12
Facial Cleansers

Facial cleansers are a cornerstone of an effective acne treatment routine. They work by removing impurities, excess oils, and dead skin cells that can clog pores and contribute to acne outbreaks. In this section, we present a collection of natural and effective facial cleansers formulated to address the unique needs of acne-prone skin.

Our recipes incorporate essential oils known for their antibacterial, anti-inflammatory, and soothing properties and other natural ingredients that cleanse and purify the skin.

These cleansers are designed to gently yet thoroughly cleanse without stripping the skin of its natural moisture. Integrating these homemade cleansers into your daily routine can help maintain a clear complexion while avoiding harsh chemicals and artificial additives.

From soothing aloe vera-based cleansers to invigorating tea tree oil formulations, these recipes offer various options tailored to different skin types and concerns. Each cleanser aims to balance and refresh the skin, providing a clean slate for further treatments and helping to prevent and manage acne more effectively. Each recipe is tailored to harness the benefits of essential oils and natural ingredients to help manage and improve acne-prone skin.

Jojoba and Green Tea Facial Cleanser

This gentle cleanser blends jojoba oil and green tea to remove impurities, balance oil production, and soothe irritation, making it perfect for maintaining clear, acne-prone skin.

What You Will Need:

- 1 tablespoon Jojoba oil
- 1 tablespoon brewed Green Tea (cooled)
- 2 drops of Tea Tree essential oil
- Small bowl
- Cotton pads

What To Do:

1. Combine the jojoba oil and green tea in a small bowl.
2. Add the tea tree oil and mix well.
3. Apply to your face using a cotton pad or your fingers.
4. Rinse with warm water and pat dry.

Tea Tree Foaming Cleanser

This foaming cleanser gently purifies the skin, using the antibacterial power of tea tree to help reduce breakouts and cleanse pores.

What You Will Need:

- 1/4 cup Liquid Castile soap
- 1/4 cup Distilled water
- 10 drops Tea Tree essential oil
- 5 drops Lavender essential oil
- Foaming pump bottle
- Mixing bowl (optional for combining)

What To Do:

1. Combine all ingredients in a foaming pump bottle.
2. Shake gently to mix.
3. Pump a small amount onto a wet face, massage in circular motions, and rinse with lukewarm water.

Aloe Vera and Chamomile Cleanser

This soothing cleanser combines aloe vera and chamomile to calm irritated skin while gently removing impurities and reducing redness.

What You Will Need:

- 1/4 cup Aloe Vera gel
- 1/4 cup Distilled water
- 5 drops Roman Chamomile essential oil
- 5 drops Tea Tree essential oil
- Pump bottle
- Mixing bowl
- Whisk or spoon

What To Do:

1. Mix aloe vera gel and distilled water in a bowl.
2. Add essential oils and stir well. Transfer to a pump bottle.
3. To use, apply to a wet face and then rinse thoroughly.

Honey and Lemon Cleanser

This brightening cleanser uses honey and lemon to cleanse pores, reduce excess oil, and promote a clearer, more radiant complexion.

What You Will Need:

- 2 tablespoons Honey
- 1 tablespoon Lemon juice
- 5 drops Lemon essential oil
- 5 drops Eucalyptus essential oil
- Mixing bowl
- Storage jar or bottle

What To Do:

1. Combine honey and lemon juice in a bowl.
2. Add essential oils and mix thoroughly.
3. Apply to damp skin, massage gently, and rinse with warm water.

Green Tea and Peppermint Cleanser

This refreshing cleanser combines green tea and peppermint to soothe the skin, reduce redness, and help clear acne.

What You Will Need:

- 1/4 cup Brewed Green Tea (cooled)
- 1/4 cup Liquid Castile soap
- 5 drops Peppermint essential oil
- 5 drops Lavender essential oil
- Bottle
- Mixing bowl (for brewing and cooling tea)

What To Do:

1. Combine green tea and castile soap in a bottle.
2. Add essential oils and shake well.
3. Use on a wet face, massage gently, and rinse thoroughly.

Yogurt and Honey Cleanser

This gentle cleanser uses yogurt and honey to moisturize the skin while helping to reduce acne and promote a clear complexion.

What You Will Need:

- 2 tablespoons Plain Yogurt
- 1 tablespoon Honey
- 5 drops Tea Tree essential oil
- 5 drops Geranium essential oil
- Mixing bowl
- Storage jar or container

What To Do:

1. Mix yogurt and honey in a bowl.
2. Add essential oils and stir well.
3. Apply to damp skin, leave on for 1-2 minutes, then rinse off with lukewarm water.

Coconut Oil and Frankincense Cleanser

This cleanser combines coconut oil and frankincense to deeply nourish and cleanse the skin, helping to reduce acne and improve skin texture.

What You Will Need:

- 2 tablespoons Coconut oil
- 1 tablespoon Liquid Castile soap
- 5 drops Frankincense essential oil
- 5 drops Myrrh essential oil
- Mixing bowl
- Container for melted oil
- Pump or squeeze bottle

What To Do:

1. Melt coconut oil if solid, then mix with castile soap in a bowl.
2. Add essential oils and blend well.
3. Apply to a wet face, massage gently, and rinse thoroughly.

Rose Water and Jojoba Cleanser

This cleanser blends rose water and jojoba oil to gently cleanse and hydrate the skin while balancing oil production and soothing inflammation.

What You Will Need:

- 1/4 cup Rose Water
- 1/4 cup Jojoba oil
- 5 drops Lavender essential oil
- 5 drops Carrot Seed essential oil
- Bottle
- Mixing bowl (optional for combining)

What To Do:

1. Combine rose water and jojoba oil in a bottle.
2. Add essential oils and shake gently.
3. Use on a wet face, massage in circular motions, and rinse well.

Apple Cider Vinegar and Tea Tree Cleanser

An apple cider vinegar and tea tree cleanser combines the clarifying properties of apple cider vinegar with the antibacterial benefits of tea tree oil to effectively cleanse and purify the skin. This formula helps remove excess oil, unclog pores, and combat acne while keeping the skin refreshed and balanced.

What You Will Need:

- 2 tablespoons Apple Cider Vinegar
- 2 tablespoons Distilled water
- 5 drops Tea Tree essential oil
- 5 drops Eucalyptus essential oil
- Bottle
- Mixing bowl (for blending)

What To Do:

1. Mix apple cider vinegar and distilled water in a bottle.
2. Add essential oils and shake well.
3. Apply to a wet face, gently massage, and rinse with lukewarm water.

Bentonite Clay and Lavender Cleanser

A bentonite clay and lavender cleanser harnesses the absorbent properties of bentonite clay to draw out impurities and excess oil, while lavender oil provides soothing and calming effects. This combination helps to purify and refresh the skin, making it ideal for balancing acne-prone skin and reducing irritation.

What You Will Need:

- 2 tablespoons Bentonite Clay
- 1/4 cup Distilled water
- 5 drops Lavender essential oil
- 5 drops Lemon essential oil
- Non-metallic bowl (bentonite clay reacts with metal)
- Application brush or fingers
- Storage jar

What To Do:

1. Mix bentonite clay with distilled water in a non-metallic bowl until smooth.
2. Add essential oils and stir well.
3. Apply to a damp face, leave on for 5-10 minutes, and rinse off with warm water.

Gentle Tea Tree Cleanser

A gentle tea tree cleanser helps to purify and refresh the skin with the antibacterial benefits of tea tree. This cleanser effectively targets acne-causing bacteria while soothing and calming the skin, making it suitable for daily use to maintain clear and healthy skin.

What You Will Need:

- 1/4 cup Castile soap
- 1/4 cup Distilled water
- 10 drops Tea Tree essential oil
- 5 drops Lavender essential oil
- 1 tablespoon Aloe Vera gel
- Small mixing bowl
- Measuring cups
- Spoon for mixing
- 4 oz bottle with pump

What To Do:

1. In a small mixing bowl, combine the castile soap and distilled water.
2. Add the aloe vera gel and essential oils. Stir well to mix.
3. Pour the mixture into a 4 oz pump bottle.
4. Use a small amount to cleanse your face, then rinse thoroughly with water.

Clarifying Lemon Cleanser

A clarifying lemon cleanser brightens the skin and helps to balance oil production. Lemon's natural astringent and antibacterial properties reduce excess oil, clear impurities, and promote a more even skin tone, making it an effective option for acne-prone skin.

What You Will Need:

- 1/4 cup Unscented liquid soap
- 1/4 cup Distilled water
- 10 drops Lemon essential oil
- 5 drops Eucalyptus essential oil
- 1 tablespoon Honey
- Small mixing bowl
- Measuring cups
- Spoon for mixing
- 4 oz bottle with pump

What To Do:

1. In a mixing bowl, combine all ingredients and stir well.
2. Pour the mixture into a 4 oz pump bottle.
3. Apply a small amount to damp skin, gently massage, and rinse with water.

Purifying Charcoal Cleanser

A purifying charcoal cleanser helps to deeply cleanse the skin by drawing out impurities and toxins. Charcoal's natural absorbent properties work to unclog pores, reduce excess oil, and improve overall skin clarity, making it ideal for acne-prone and oily skin types.

What You Will Need:

- 1 tablespoon Activated Charcoal
- 1/4 cup Liquid Castile soap
- 1/4 cup Distilled water
- 8 drops Tea Tree essential oil
- 5 drops Lavender essential oil
- Small mixing bowl
- Measuring spoons
- Spoon for mixing
- 4 oz bottle with pump

What To Do:

1. Mix activated charcoal, castile soap, and distilled water in a small bowl.
2. Add essential oils and stir until well combined.
3. Transfer to a 4 oz pump bottle.
4. Use as a daily cleanser, massaging onto wet skin before rinsing.

Calming Chamomile Cleanser

A calming chamomile cleanser offers gentle yet effective cleansing while soothing the skin. Chamomile's anti-inflammatory and calming properties help reduce redness and irritation, making it an excellent choice for sensitive, acne-prone skin.

What You Will Need:

- 1/4 cup Chamomile Tea (cooled)
- 1/4 cup Liquid Castile soap
- 1 tablespoon Jojoba oil
- 8 drops Chamomile essential oil
- 5 drops Lavender essential oil
- Small mixing bowl
- Measuring cups
- Spoon for mixing
- 4 oz bottle with pump

What To Do:

1. Brew chamomile tea and let it cool completely.
2. Mix the tea with castile soap and jojoba oil in a bowl.
3. Add essential oils and stir well.
4. Pour into a 4 oz pump bottle and shake before each use.

Soothing Aloe Cleanser

A soothing aloe cleanser gently cleanses the skin while providing calming relief and hydration. Aloe vera's natural soothing properties help reduce redness and irritation, making it ideal for sensitive and acne-prone skin.

What You Will Need:

- 1/4 cup Aloe Vera gel
- 1/4 cup Liquid Castile soap
- 1/4 cup Distilled water
- 10 drops Lavender essential oil
- 5 drops Frankincense essential oil
- Small mixing bowl
- Measuring cups
- Spoon for mixing
- 4 oz bottle with pump

What To Do:

1. Combine aloe vera gel, castile soap, and distilled water in a mixing bowl.
2. Add essential oils and stir until well blended.
3. Pour into a 4 oz pump bottle and shake before each use.

Refreshing Peppermint Cleanser

A refreshing peppermint cleanser invigorates the skin with a cooling sensation while effectively removing impurities and excess oil. Its peppermint essence stimulates and refreshes the complexion, leaving it clean and revitalized.

What You Will Need:

- 1/4 cup Liquid Castile soap
- 1/4 cup Distilled water
- 8 drops Peppermint essential oil
- 5 drops Tea Tree essential oil
- 1 tablespoon Witch Hazel
- Small mixing bowl
- Measuring cups
- Spoon for mixing
- 4 oz bottle with pump

What To Do:

1. Mix the castile soap and distilled water in a small bowl.
2. Add witch hazel and essential oils, stirring well.
3. Pour into a 4 oz pump bottle and shake before each use.

Hydrating Coconut Cleanser

A hydrating coconut cleanser utilizes the moisturizing properties of coconut to gently cleanse and nourish the skin, providing essential hydration while removing impurities for a soft, supple, and refreshed complexion.

What You Will Need:

- 1/4 cup Fractionated Coconut oil
- 1/4 cup Liquid Castile soap
- 1/4 cup Distilled water
- 8 drops Lavender essential oil
- 5 drops Geranium essential oil
- Small mixing bowl
- Measuring cups
- Spoon for mixing
- 4 oz bottle with pump

What To Do:

1. Combine fractionated coconut oil, castile soap, and distilled water in a mixing bowl.
2. Add essential oils and stir until well blended.
3. Transfer to a 4 oz pump bottle and shake before use.

Detoxifying Green Tea Cleanser

A detoxifying green tea cleanser harnesses the antioxidant power of green tea to cleanse and purify the skin, helping to remove toxins and excess oil while soothing and rejuvenating the complexion for a fresh, healthy appearance.

What You Will Need:

- 1/4 cup Brewed Green Tea (cooled)
- 1/4 cup Liquid Castile soap
- 1 tablespoon Aloe Vera gel
- 8 drops Tea Tree essential oil
- 5 drops Lemon essential oil
- Small mixing bowl
- Measuring cups
- Spoon for mixing
- 4 oz bottle with pump

What To Do:

1. Brew green tea and let it cool completely.
2. Mix the tea with castile soap and aloe vera gel in a bowl.
3. Add essential oils and stir well.
4. Pour into a 4 oz pump bottle and shake before each use.

Gentle Rose Cleanser

A gentle rose cleanser uses the soothing and hydrating properties of rose essential oil to calm and refresh the skin while effectively removing impurities, leaving the complexion soft, balanced, and revitalized.

What You Will Need:

- 1/4 cup Rose Water
- 1/4 cup Liquid Castile soap
- 1 tablespoon Jojoba oil
- 8 drops Rose essential oil
- 5 drops Frankincense essential oil
- Small mixing bowl
- Measuring cups
- Spoon for mixing
- 4 oz bottle with pump

What To Do:

1. Combine rose water, castile soap, and jojoba oil in a mixing bowl.
2. Add essential oils and stir until well blended.
3. Transfer to a 4 oz pump bottle and shake before use.

Brightening Citrus Cleanser

A brightening citrus cleanser combines the stimulating properties of citrus essential oils to refresh and illuminate the skin. It gently cleanses impurities and excess oil, making it ideal for achieving a radiant complexion.

What You Will Need:

- 1/4 cup Liquid Castile soap
- 1/4 cup Distilled water
- 8 drops Lemon essential oil
- 5 drops Grapefruit essential oil
- 1 tablespoon Honey
- Small mixing bowl
- Measuring cups
- Spoon for mixing
- 4 oz bottle with pump

What To Do:

1. Mix castile soap, distilled water, and honey in a small bowl.
2. Add essential oils and stir well.
3. Pour into a 4 oz pump bottle and shake before each use.

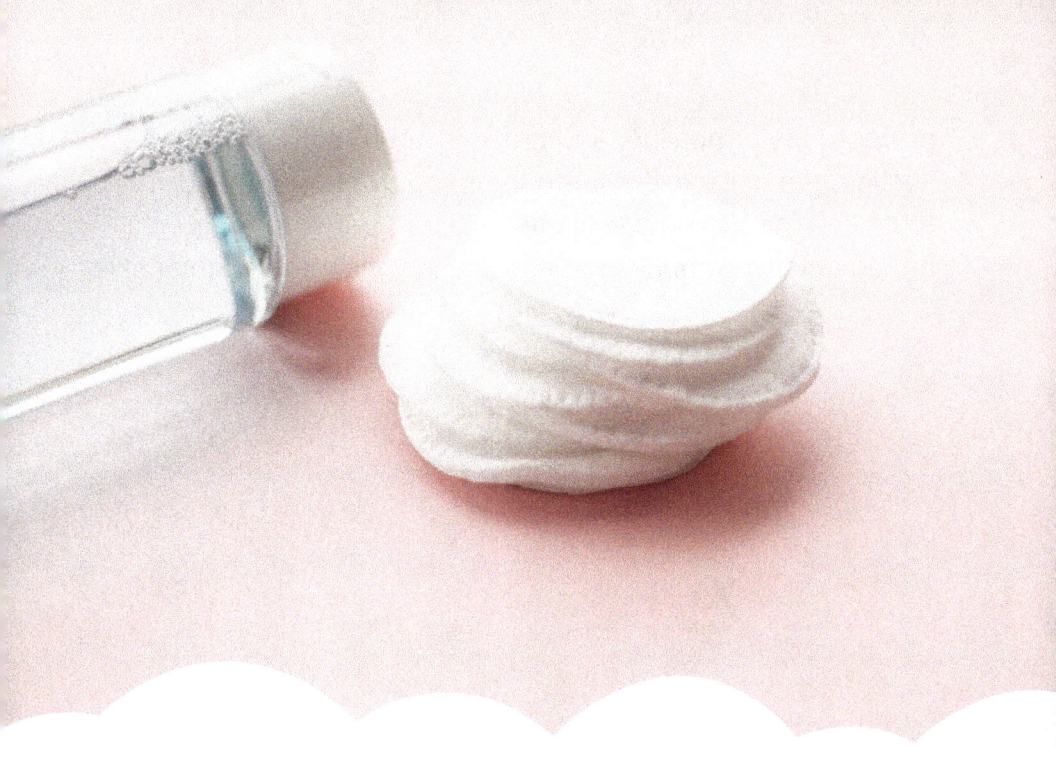

Chapter 13
Spot Treatments

Acne can be persistent and unpredictable, often manifesting as unexpected breakouts requiring targeted intervention. Spot treatments offer a focused approach to managing these localized blemishes, delivering concentrated ingredients directly to the problem areas. These treatments are designed to address the underlying causes of acne, such as excess oil, bacteria, and inflammation, with precision and effectiveness. By using essential oils and natural ingredients known for their antibacterial, anti-inflammatory, and soothing properties, spot treatments can help reduce the size and redness of pimples, promote faster healing, and prevent future outbreaks. In this section, we will explore a range of spot treatment recipes that combine the power of essential oils with other potent ingredients to combat acne and support clearer, healthier skin.

Honey and Cinnamon Spot Treatment

Honey and cinnamon spot treatment leverages honey's natural antibacterial properties and cinnamon's anti-inflammatory benefits to reduce the appearance of acne spots, helping to soothe the skin and accelerate healing.

What You Will Need:

- 1 tablespoon Honey
- 1/2 teaspoon Ground Cinnamon
- 2 drops of Tea Tree essential oil

What To Do:

1. Combine the honey and ground cinnamon in a bowl.
2. Add the tea tree oil and mix well.
3. Apply directly to blemishes and leave on for 10-15 minutes.
4. Rinse off with warm water.

Tea Tree Spot Treatment

Tea tree spot treatment targets acne spots with its potent antibacterial and anti-inflammatory properties, helping reduce blemishes' size and redness while preventing future breakouts.

What You Will Need:

- 1 teaspoon Tea Tree essential oil
- 1 teaspoon Aloe Vera gel
- Small mixing bowl
- Cotton swab

What To Do:

1. Mix the tea tree and aloe vera gel in a small container.
2. Apply directly to the affected area using a cotton swab.
3. Leave on for 15-20 minutes, then rinse off with lukewarm water.

Lavender and Frankincense Spot Treatment

This spot treatment combines lavender and frankincense essential oils to harness their calming and healing properties, aiming to soothe irritated skin and reduce the appearance of blemishes while promoting overall skin repair and rejuvenation.

What You Will Need:

- 1 teaspoon Lavender essential oil
- 1 teaspoon Frankincense essential oil
- 1 teaspoon Jojoba oil
- Small mixing bowl
- Cotton swab

What To Do:

1. Combine the lavender, frankincense, and jojoba oils in a small container.
2. Gently dab onto the blemish using a cotton swab or clean fingertip.
3. Leave overnight and rinse off in the morning.

Peppermint and Lemon Spot Treatment

This spot treatment blends peppermint and lemon essential oils to leverage their antimicrobial and astringent properties, targeting blemishes with a cooling effect and helping to reduce redness and oiliness for a more balanced complexion.

What You Will Need:

- 1 teaspoon Peppermint essential oil
- 1 teaspoon Lemon essential oil
- 1 teaspoon Witch Hazel
- Small mixing bowl
- Cotton swab

What To Do:

1. Mix the peppermint, lemon, and witch hazel in a small container.
2. Apply directly to the pimple with a cotton swab.
3. Allow to dry before applying any other products.

Green Tea and Tea Tree Spot Treatment

This spot treatment combines green tea and tea tree oil to harness their anti-inflammatory and antibacterial properties. It provides a dual-action approach to soothe irritated skin and combat acne-causing bacteria for clearer, healthier skin.

What You Will Need:

- 1 tablespoon Brewed Green Tea (cooled)
- 1 teaspoon Tea Tree essential oil
- 1 teaspoon Aloe Vera gel
- Small mixing bowl
- Cotton swab

What To Do:

1. Combine the brewed green tea, tea tree oil, and aloe vera gel in a small container.
2. Apply to the blemish with a cotton swab.
3. Leave on for 15 minutes and then rinse off with lukewarm water.

Benzoyl Peroxide and Eucalyptus Spot Treatment

This spot treatment blends benzoyl peroxide with eucalyptus oil to effectively combat acne by targeting bacteria and reducing inflammation, offering a potent solution for treating individual blemishes and preventing future breakouts.

What You Will Need:

- 1 teaspoon Benzoyl Peroxide (2.5% or 5%)
- 3 drops Eucalyptus essential oil
- Small mixing bowl
- Cotton swab

What To Do:

1. Mix the benzoyl peroxide and eucalyptus oil in a small bowl.
2. Apply to the affected area with a clean fingertip or cotton swab.
3. Leave overnight and wash off in the morning.

Clove Bud and Geranium Spot Treatment

This spot treatment combines clove bud and geranium oils to target acne with their antibacterial and anti-inflammatory properties, helping to reduce blemishes and soothe irritated skin while promoting a clearer complexion.

What You Will Need:

- 1 teaspoon Clove Bud essential oil
- 1 teaspoon Geranium essential oil
- 1 teaspoon Fractionated Coconut oil
- Small mixing bowl
- Cotton swab

What To Do:

1. Blend the clove bud, geranium, and fractionated coconut oils in a small container.
2. Dab onto the spot using a cotton swab.
3. Leave it on overnight and rinse it off in the morning.

Chamomile and Rosehip Seed Oil Spot Treatment

This spot treatment harnesses the soothing and healing properties of chamomile and rosehip seed oil to calm irritated skin and promote faster healing of blemishes while reducing redness and inflammation.

What You Will Need:

- 1 teaspoon Chamomile essential oil
- 1 teaspoon Rosehip Seed oil
- Small mixing bowl
- Cotton swab

What To Do:

1. Mix the chamomile and rosehip seed oils in a small bowl.
2. Apply to the blemish using a clean fingertip or cotton swab.
3. Let it sit for 20 minutes before rinsing off with lukewarm water.

Myrrh and Witch Hazel Spot Treatment

Combining myrrh with witch hazel, this spot treatment helps reduce the appearance of blemishes by offering anti-inflammatory and astringent properties, promoting clearer skin and faster recovery.

What You Will Need:

- 1 teaspoon Myrrh essential oil
- 1 teaspoon Witch Hazel
- 1 teaspoon Aloe Vera gel
- Small mixing bowl
- Cotton swab

What To Do:

1. Combine the myrrh, witch hazel, and aloe vera gel in a small container.
2. Apply to the affected area with a cotton swab.
3. Leave on for 10-15 minutes and rinse with lukewarm water.

Carrot Seed and Lavender Spot Treatment

This spot treatment blends carrot seed oil with lavender to target blemishes, reducing inflammation and promoting faster healing while soothing the skin.

What You Will Need:

- 1 teaspoon Carrot Seed essential oil
- 1 teaspoon Lavender essential oil
- 1 teaspoon Jojoba oil
- Small mixing bowl
- Cotton swab

What To Do:

1. Blend the carrot seed, lavender, and jojoba oils in a small bowl.
2. Dab onto the pimple using a clean fingertip or cotton swab.
3. Allow to absorb overnight and wash off in the morning.

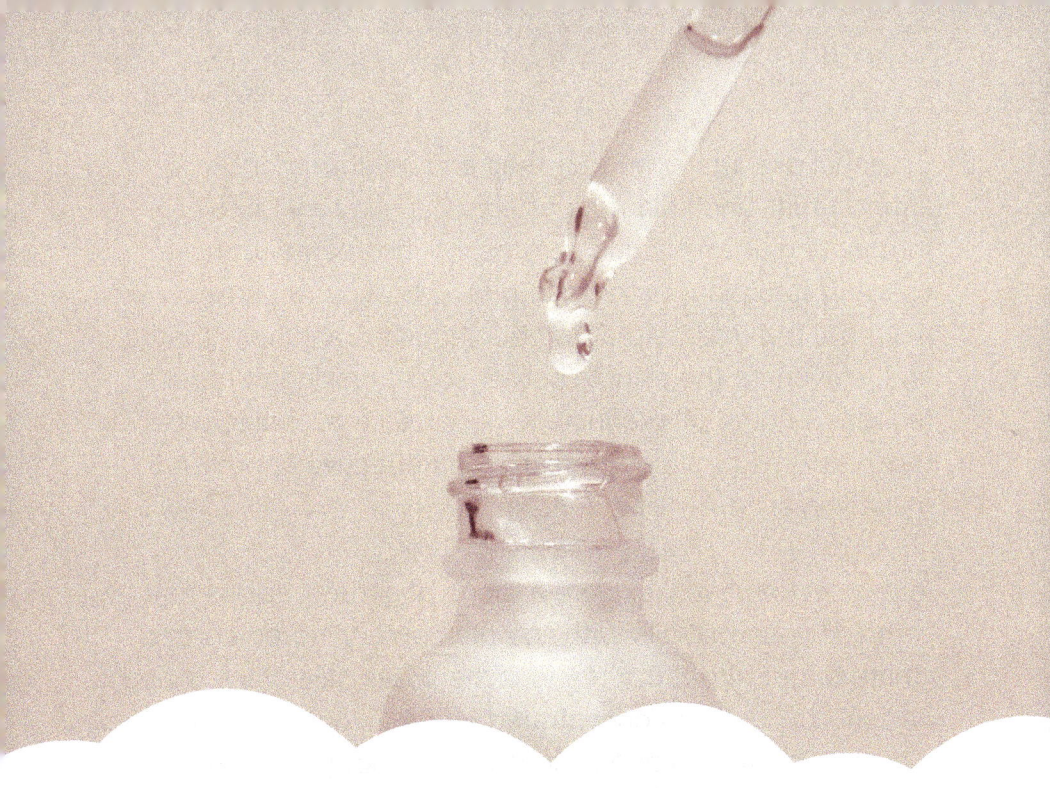

Chapter 14
Serums

In the quest for clear, healthy skin, serums are potent for targeting acne and enhancing your skincare routine. Unlike traditional cleansers and moisturizers, serums are formulated with a higher concentration of active ingredients, allowing them to penetrate deeper into the skin and address specific concerns more effectively. When tailored with essential oils, these serums can harness the therapeutic properties of nature to combat acne, reduce inflammation, and promote healing.

Essential oils, renowned for their anti-inflammatory, antibacterial, and balancing effects, can play a vital role in formulating acne-fighting serums. By incorporating these concentrated plant extracts into serums, you can create powerful treatments that target blemishes and help soothe and rejuvenate the skin. Whether you're looking to reduce redness, control oil production, or enhance overall skin clarity, these serums provide a versatile and effective approach to managing acne.

In this section, we'll explore a range of serum recipes that combine essential oils with complementary ingredients to create targeted treatments for acne-prone skin. Each recipe is designed to deliver concentrated benefits, helping you achieve a clearer, healthier complexion with the power of nature.

Serums are a powerful addition to any skincare routine, offering concentrated ingredients that penetrate deeply to target specific skin concerns. For those struggling with acne, serums can be particularly effective, delivering potent anti-inflammatory, antibacterial, and healing properties directly to the skin. Unlike heavier creams or lotions, serums are lightweight and easily absorbed, making them ideal for treating acne without clogging pores or leaving a greasy residue. In this section, you'll find a selection of serum recipes crafted with essential oils known for their acne-fighting abilities. These blends help reduce blemishes, prevent future breakouts, and nourish and soothe the skin, promoting a clearer, healthier complexion. Whether used as part of your morning or evening routine, these serums provide a natural, effective way to combat acne and restore your skin's balance.

Rosehip and Green Tea Serum

This serum combines rosehip seed oil and green tea to nourish and rejuvenate the skin, offering antioxidant protection and promoting a clear, healthy complexion. Use this serum as part of your nightly skincare routine to benefit from its soothing and rejuvenating properties.

What You Will Need:

- 1 tablespoon Rosehip Seed oil
- 1 tablespoon Brewed Green Tea (cooled)
- 3 drops Lavender essential oil
- Small dropper bottle (1 oz or 30 ml)
- Small bowl or measuring cup
- Stirring tool (e.g., small spoon or dropper)
- Strainer (if brewing green tea)

What To Do:

1. Brew a small amount of green tea and let it cool completely—strain to remove any leaves if necessary.
2. Mix the cooled green tea and rosehip seed oil in a small bowl or measuring cup.
3. Transfer the mixture to a small dropper bottle using a funnel if needed. Add the lavender essential oil.
4. Secure the cap and shake the bottle gently to blend the oils thoroughly.
5. Apply a few drops of the serum to your face and gently massage it using upward motions.

Tea Tree and Jojoba Serum

A tea tree and jojoba serum offers a potent combination of tea tree oil's antibacterial properties and jojoba oil's moisturizing benefits. This serum helps reduce acne-causing bacteria, soothe inflammation, and maintain the skin's natural moisture balance, making it ideal for those with acne-prone skin seeking treatment and hydration.

What You Will Need:

- 1 tablespoon Jojoba oil
- 5 drops Tea Tree essential oil
- 3 drops Lavender essential oil
- Small dropper bottle (1 oz or 30 ml)
- Small bowl or measuring cup
- Stirring tool (e.g., small spoon or dropper)

What To Do:

1. Combine jojoba, tea tree, and lavender oil in a small bowl.
2. Transfer the mixture to a small dropper bottle.
3. Secure the cap and shake gently to blend.
4. Apply a few drops to acne-prone areas and gently massage in.

Frankincense and Argan Serum

This frankincense, argan, and geranium serum combines the anti-inflammatory and rejuvenating properties of frankincense with the nourishing benefits of argan oil and the balancing effects of geranium. This serum helps reduce redness and inflammation, promotes skin healing, and provides deep hydration, making it ideal for calming and restoring acne-prone skin.

What You Will Need:

- 1 tablespoon Argan oil
- 4 drops Frankincense essential oil
- 3 drops Geranium essential oil
- Small dropper bottle (1 oz or 30 ml)
- Small bowl or measuring cup
- Stirring tool

What To Do:

1. Combine argan, frankincense, and geranium in a small bowl.
2. Transfer the mixture to a small dropper bottle.
3. Secure the cap and shake gently to blend.
4. Apply a few drops to your face and gently massage in.

Rosehip and Chamomile Serum

This serum blends the skin-rejuvenating properties of rosehip oil with the soothing effects of chamomile and the healing benefits of helichrysum. This serum helps reduce redness, improve skin texture, and promote overall skin healing, making it a calming and restorative choice for acne-prone or sensitive skin.

What You Will Need:

- 1 tablespoon Rosehip Seed oil
- 3 drops Roman Chamomile essential oil
- 3 drops Helichrysum essential oil
- Small dropper bottle (1 oz or 30 ml)
- Small bowl or measuring cup
- Stirring tool

What To Do:

1. Combine rosehip seed, chamomile, and helichrysum oil in a small bowl.
2. Transfer the mixture to a small dropper bottle.
3. Secure the cap and shake gently to blend.
4. Apply a few drops to your face and gently massage in.

Lavender and Grapeseed Serum

A lavender, tea tree, and grapeseed serum combines the calming and antibacterial properties of lavender and tea tree oils with the moisturizing benefits of grapeseed oil. This serum targets acne while soothing inflammation, balancing oil production, and hydrating the skin. It's ideal for promoting clearer, more balanced, and hydrated skin.

What You Will Need:

- 1 tablespoon Grapeseed oil
- 4 drops Lavender essential oil
- 3 drops Tea Tree essential oil
- Small dropper bottle (1 oz or 30 ml)
- Small bowl or measuring cup
- Stirring tool

What To Do:

1. Combine grapeseed, lavender, and tea tree oil in a small bowl.
2. Transfer the mixture to a small dropper bottle.
3. Secure the cap and shake gently to blend.
4. Apply a few drops to your face and gently massage in.

Aloe Vera and Sandalwood Serum

An aloe vera and sandalwood serum combines the soothing and hydrating properties of aloe vera with the anti-inflammatory and calming benefits of sandalwood. This serum is designed to calm irritated skin, reduce redness, and provide deep hydration, making it ideal for soothing acne-prone and sensitive skin.

What You Will Need:

- 1 tablespoon Aloe Vera gel
- 4 drops Sandalwood essential oil
- 3 drops Lavender essential oil
- Small dropper bottle (1 oz or 30 ml)
- Small bowl or measuring cup
- Stirring tool

What To Do:

1. Combine aloe vera gel, sandalwood, and lavender oil in a small bowl.
2. Transfer the mixture to a small dropper bottle.
3. Secure the cap and shake gently to blend.
4. Apply a few drops to your face and gently massage in.

Clary Sage and Hemp Seed Serum

Combining clary sage with hemp seed oil balances oil production, soothes inflammation, and hydrates the skin. It is an excellent choice for managing acne-prone and oily skin while promoting overall skin health.

What You Will Need:

- 1 tablespoon Hemp Seed oil
- 4 drops Clary Sage essential oil
- 3 drops Tea Tree essential oil
- Small dropper bottle (1 oz or 30 ml)
- Small bowl or measuring cup
- Stirring tool

What To Do:

1. Combine hemp seed, clary sage, and tea tree oils in a small bowl.
2. Transfer the mixture to a small dropper bottle.
3. Secure the cap and shake gently to blend.
4. Apply a few drops to your face and gently massage in.

Calendula and Neroli Serum

Blending calendula with neroli oil helps to calm irritated skin, promote healing, and improve skin tone, making it beneficial for sensitive and acne-prone skin.

What You Will Need:

- 1 tablespoon Calendula oil
- 4 drops Neroli essential oil
- 3 drops Lavender essential oil
- Small dropper bottle (1 oz or 30 ml)
- Small bowl or measuring cup
- Stirring tool

What To Do:

1. Combine calendula, neroli, and lavender oils in a small bowl.
2. Transfer the mixture to a small dropper bottle.
3. Secure the cap and shake gently to blend.
4. Apply a few drops to your face and gently massage in.

Tamanu and Geranium Serum

Combining tamanu with geranium oils supports skin regeneration and balances oil production, which can be particularly helpful for treating acne and reducing the appearance of scars.

What You Will Need:

- 1 tablespoon Tamanu oil
- 4 drops Geranium essential oil
- 3 drops Tea Tree essential oil
- Small dropper bottle (1 oz or 30 ml)
- Small bowl or measuring cup
- Stirring tool

What To Do:

1. Combine tamanu, geranium, and tea tree oils in a small bowl.
2. Transfer the mixture to a small dropper bottle.
3. Secure the cap and shake gently to blend.
4. Apply a few drops to your face and gently massage in.

Neem and Rosemary Serum

Using neem and rosemary oils together provides antibacterial and anti-inflammatory benefits, helping to cleanse the skin and reduce acne breakouts while promoting a clearer complexion.

What You Will Need:

- 1 tablespoon Neem oil
- 4 drops Rosemary essential oil
- 3 drops Tea Tree essential oil
- Small dropper bottle (1 oz or 30 ml)
- Small bowl or measuring cup
- Stirring tool

What To Do:

1. Combine neem, rosemary, and tea tree oils in a small bowl.
2. Transfer the mixture to a small dropper bottle.
3. Secure the cap and shake gently to blend.
4. Apply a few drops to your face and gently massage in.

Balancing Acne Serum

A carefully formulated blend designed to balance oil production, reduce breakouts, and soothe inflammation, promoting healthier and clearer skin.

What You Will Need:

- 10 drops Clary Sage essential oil
- 10 drops Tea Tree essential oil
- 5 drops Carrot Seed essential oil
- 2 tablespoons Rosehip Seed oil
- Small funnel
- 1 oz glass dropper bottle
- Measuring spoons

What To Do:

1. Place the small funnel over the mouth of the dropper bottle.
2. Add the clary sage, tea tree, and carrot seed oils into the funnel, followed by the rosehip seed oil.
3. Remove the funnel and securely close the dropper bottle. Shake well to ensure the oils are thoroughly combined.
4. Apply a few drops to clean skin before bedtime, focusing on acne-prone areas.

Hydrating Acne Serum

A lightweight serum that provides deep hydration while targeting acne, helping to keep skin moisturized and clear without clogging pores.

What You Will Need:

- 5 drops Geranium essential oil
- 5 drops Lavender essential oil
- 5 drops Frankincense essential oil
- 2 tablespoons Argan oil
- Small funnel
- 1 oz Glass dropper bottle
- Measuring spoons

What To Do:

1. Set up the funnel over the dropper bottle.
2. Pour the geranium, lavender, and frankincense oils into the bottle, followed by the argan oil.
3. Remove the funnel and close the bottle tightly. Shake well to mix the ingredients.
4. Use a few drops on clean skin, particularly on areas prone to dryness, either morning or evening.

Clarifying Anti-Acne Serum

This potent serum helps to clarify the skin by reducing excess oil and targeting acne, promoting a clearer and more balanced complexion.

What You Will Need:

- 8 drops Lavender essential oil
- 8 drops Tea Tree essential oil
- 4 drops Lemon essential oil
- 2 tablespoons Jojoba oil
- Small funnel
- 1 oz glass dropper bottle
- Measuring spoons

What To Do:

1. Use the funnel to add the essential oils and jojoba oil to the dropper bottle.
2. Shake well before each use. Apply a few drops to the face, focusing on acne-prone areas.

Soothing Redness Serum

A calming serum that helps reduce redness and irritation, soothing sensitive acne-prone skin for a more even complexion.

What You Will Need:

- 7 drops Roman Chamomile essential oil
- 7 drops Helichrysum essential oil
- 6 drops Lavender essential oil
- 2 tablespoons Sweet Almond oil
- Small funnel
- 1 oz glass dropper bottle
- Measuring spoons

What To Do:

1. Using the funnel, combine the essential oils with almond oil in the dropper bottle.
2. Shake well and apply to areas with redness or inflammation.

Anti-Inflammatory Acne Serum

A targeted serum designed to reduce inflammation and calm irritated skin, aiding in treating acne.

What You Will Need:

- 8 drops Blue Tansy essential oil
- 6 drops Frankincense essential oil
- 6 drops Lavender essential oil
- 2 tablespoons Grapeseed oil
- Small funnel
- 1 oz glass dropper bottle
- Measuring spoons

What To Do:

1. Pour the essential and grapeseed oils into the dropper bottle using the funnel.
2. Shake to combine. Apply to inflamed or irritated skin as needed.

Nourishing Night Serum

This deep moisturizing serum is formulated to rejuvenate and repair the skin overnight, promoting a clearer complexion and reducing the appearance of acne.

What You Will Need:

- 8 drops Rose essential oil
- 8 drops Myrrh essential oil
- 4 drops Neroli essential oil
- 2 tablespoons Evening Primrose oil
- Small funnel
- 1 oz glass dropper bottle
- Measuring spoons

What To Do:

1. Using the funnel, add the essential oils and evening primrose oil to the dropper bottle.
2. Shake well and apply before bed to nourish and rejuvenate the skin.

Brightening Acne Serum

This serum is designed to enhance skin radiance and even out skin tone while targeting acne spots and scars for a brighter, clearer complexion.

What You Will Need:

- 10 drops Carrot Seed essential oil
- 5 drops Lemon essential oil
- 5 drops Frankincense essential oil
- 2 tablespoons Rosehip Seed oil
- Small funnel
- 1 oz glass dropper bottle
- Measuring spoons

What To Do:

1. Combine all ingredients in the dropper bottle using the funnel.
2. Shake well before each use and apply in the morning for a brighter complexion.

Blemish-Fighting Serum

A blemish-fighting serum effectively reduces and prevents acne by targeting the key factors contributing to breakouts.

What You Will Need:

- 10 drops Tea Tree essential oil
- 5 drops Lavender essential oil
- 5 drops Patchouli essential oil
- 2 tablespoons Tamanu oil
- Small funnel
- 1 oz glass dropper bottle
- Measuring spoons

What To Do:

1. Use the funnel to add all oils into the dropper bottle.
2. Shake well to combine. Apply to blemishes at night.

Skin-Balancing Serum

A skin-balancing serum effectively achieves a harmonious complexion by regulating the skin's oil production and improving its overall texture. This serum typically combines essential oils and active ingredients that balance sebum levels, reduce excess oil, and address dryness or dehydration. Using this serum regularly helps maintain an optimal skin environment, reducing the likelihood of breakouts and promoting a smoother, more even-toned appearance.

What You Will Need:

- 10 drops Geranium essential oil
- 5 drops Ylang Ylang essential oil
- 5 drops Sandalwood essential oil
- 2 tablespoons Marula oil
- Small funnel
- 1 oz glass dropper bottle
- Measuring spoons

What To Do:

1. Add essential oils and marula oil to the dropper bottle using the funnel.
2. Shake well and apply to the face, focusing on areas where oil production needs balancing.

Healing Acne Scar Serum

A healing acne scar serum using helichrysum and lavender essential oils promotes the repair and regeneration of skin affected by acne scars. This type of serum leverages the regenerative properties of essential oils such as rosehip seed oil and helichrysum to stimulate collagen production, improve skin texture, and reduce the appearance of scars. The blend of these oils helps to soothe inflammation, lighten dark spots, and accelerate healing, leading to a more even and rejuvenated skin surface. Regularly using this serum can help fade scars and improve the skin's overall appearance.

What You Will Need:

- 8 drops Helichrysum essential oil
- 8 drops Rosehip Seed oil
- 4 drops Lavender essential oil
- 2 tablespoons Tamanu oil
- Small funnel
- 1 oz glass dropper bottle
- Measuring spoons

What To Do:

1. Pour all ingredients into the dropper bottle using the funnel.
2. Shake well before each use. Apply to acne scars to promote healing and reduce their appearance.

Gentle Acne Serum

A gentle acne serum formulated with essential oils addresses acne concerns without causing irritation or excessive dryness. This serum typically features soothing oils, such as chamomile and lavender, combined with balancing oils like jojoba or rosehip seed oil. The blend reduces inflammation, controls excess oil, and promotes healing while maintaining the skin's natural moisture balance. Ideal for sensitive skin, this serum helps to prevent breakouts and supports a clearer, healthier complexion while being kind to the skin.

What You Will Need:

- 8 drops Chamomile essential oil
- 6 drops Lavender essential oil
- 6 drops Frankincense essential oil
- 2 tablespoons Jojoba oil
- Small funnel
- 1 oz glass dropper bottle
- Measuring spoons

What To Do:

1. Mix the essential oils and jojoba oil in a dropper bottle using the funnel.
2. Shake well and apply to sensitive or irritated areas to soothe and protect.

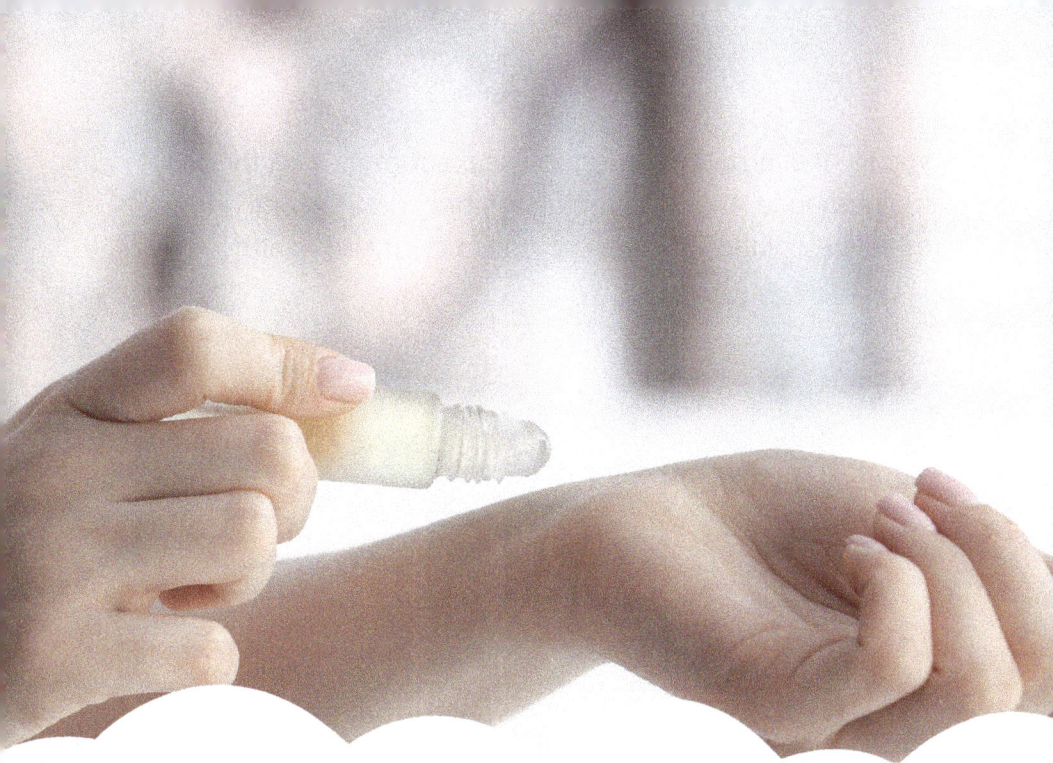

Chapter 15
Roll-On Recipes

Roll-ons are a convenient and targeted way to deliver the healing properties of essential oils directly to problem areas, making them especially effective for acne treatment. These compact, easy-to-use applicators allow for precise application, ensuring that potent ingredients reach the areas that need them most without waste. Roll-ons are perfect for on-the-go use, fitting easily into your purse or pocket, so you can treat blemishes and inflammation whenever required. In this section, you'll discover a variety of roll-on recipes designed to soothe, heal, and balance acne-prone skin. Whether you're dealing with a sudden breakout or looking for daily maintenance, these formulations provide a natural and effective solution to keep your skin clear and healthy.

Acne Spot Treatment Roll-On

An acne spot treatment roll-on is a convenient and targeted solution for addressing individual blemishes. Formulated with essential oils known for their antibacterial and anti-inflammatory properties, this treatment often includes oils like tea tree and lavender to help combat acne-causing bacteria, reduce redness, and accelerate healing. The roll-on applicator allows for precise application directly on problem areas, ensuring effective treatment without disturbing the surrounding skin. It is ideal for on-the-go use, provides quick relief, and helps prevent future breakouts.

What You Will Need:

- 10 drops Tea Tree essential oil
- 5 drops Lavender essential oil
- 5 drops Frankincense essential oil
- 2 tablespoons Jojoba oil
- 10 ml glass roll-on bottle
- Small funnel (optional)
- Measuring spoons

What To Do:

1. Add the tea tree, lavender, and frankincense oils to the roll-on bottle using a small funnel.
2. Pour in the jojoba oil using a measuring spoon, filling the rest of the bottle.
3. Secure the rollerball top and cap, then shake well to combine the ingredients.
4. Shake the bottle before each use to ensure the oils are evenly mixed.
5. Apply directly to blemishes and problem areas as needed.

Soothing Anti-Acne Roll-On

A soothing anti-acne roll-on is designed to calm irritated skin while treating breakouts. This gentle formula typically includes essential oils such as chamomile and lavender, known for their soothing and anti-inflammatory properties. The roll-on applicator allows for easy, precise application directly to blemishes, helping to reduce redness and discomfort while promoting faster healing. Perfect for sensitive or inflamed skin, this treatment offers a calming approach to acne care, helping to balance and protect the skin.

What You Will Need:

- 8 drops Roman Chamomile essential oil
- 8 drops Helichrysum essential oil
- 4 drops Geranium essential oil
- 2 tablespoons Fractionated Coconut oil
- 10 ml glass roll-on bottle
- Small funnel (optional)
- Measuring spoons

What To Do:

1. Place the Roman chamomile, helichrysum, and geranium oil into the roll-on bottle using a small funnel for precision.
2. Add the fractionated coconut oil using a measuring spoon to fill the remainder of the bottle.
3. Attach the rollerball top and cap, then shake gently to blend the oils.
4. Shake the bottle lightly before each application.
5. Apply to inflamed or irritated areas of the skin twice daily for soothing relief.

Calming Lavender and Tea Tree Roll-On

A calming roll-on with lavender and tea tree oil is ideal for addressing acne gently yet effectively. Lavender soothes irritated skin and reduces redness, while tea tree oil's antibacterial properties help to clear blemishes and prevent future breakouts. The convenient roll-on applicator makes it easy to target specific areas, providing a calming, spot-treatment solution for sensitive skin.

What You Will Need:

- 8 drops Lavender essential oil
- 7 drops Tea Tree essential oil
- 5 drops Frankincense essential oil
- 2 tablespoons Sweet Almond oil
- 10 ml glass roll-on bottle
- Small funnel (optional)
- Measuring spoons

What To Do:

1. Add lavender, tea tree, and frankincense oil to the roll-on bottle using a funnel.
2. Pour in sweet almond oil to fill the remainder of the bottle.
3. Attach the rollerball top and cap, then shake well to mix.
4. Apply directly to acne-prone areas for calming effects.

Clary Sage and Geranium Acne Roll-On

This acne roll-on combines clary sage and geranium essential oils to help balance the skin's natural oils and reduce inflammation. Clary sage helps regulate sebum production, while geranium promotes skin healing and reduces redness. The roll-on applicator provides a convenient way to apply the blend directly to acne-prone areas, offering a soothing and balancing treatment for breakouts.

What You Will Need:

- 6 drops Clary Sage essential oil
- 6 drops Geranium essential oil
- 8 drops Tea Tree essential oil
- 2 tablespoons Jojoba oil
- 10 ml glass roll-on bottle
- Small funnel (optional)
- Measuring spoons

What To Do:

1. Combine clary sage, geranium, and tea tree oils in the roll-on bottle using a funnel.
2. Add jojoba oil to fill the rest of the bottle.
3. Secure the rollerball top and cap, then shake to blend.
4. Apply to acne spots as needed for a balancing treatment.

Purifying Lemongrass and Peppermint Roll-On

This purifying roll-on blend features lemongrass and peppermint essential oils, known for their antibacterial and refreshing properties. Lemongrass helps to cleanse the skin and reduce excess oil, while peppermint provides a cooling sensation that soothes irritation and tightens pores. The roll-on format allows for easy application directly to blemishes, making it an effective spot treatment for acne-prone skin.

What You Will Need:

- 8 drops Lemongrass essential oil
- 5 drops Peppermint essential oil
- 7 drops Lavender essential oil
- 2 tablespoons Fractionated Coconut oil
- 10 ml glass roll-on bottle
- Small funnel (optional)
- Measuring spoons

What To Do:

1. Using a funnel, add lemongrass, peppermint, and lavender oil to the roll-on bottle.
2. Fill the remainder of the bottle with fractionated coconut oil.
3. Attach the rollerball top and cap, then shake to combine.
4. Roll onto affected areas to purify and refresh the skin.

Healing Rosehip and Myrrh Roll-On

This healing roll-on combines rosehip oil's regenerative properties with myrrh essential oil's soothing benefits. Rosehip oil is rich in vitamins and fatty acids that help reduce the appearance of scars and promote skin renewal, while myrrh aids in calming inflammation and supporting the skin's natural healing process. Together, they create a potent blend that targets acne scars and blemishes, promoting smoother and healthier skin.

What You Will Need:

- 6 drops Myrrh essential oil
- 6 drops Lavender essential oil
- 8 drops Tea Tree essential oil
- 2 tablespoons Rosehip Seed oil
- 10 ml glass roll-on bottle
- Small funnel (optional)
- Measuring spoons

What To Do:

1. Place myrrh, lavender, and tea tree oils into the roll-on bottle using a funnel.
2. Add rosehip seed oil to fill the remainder of the bottle.
3. Attach the rollerball top and cap, then shake well.
4. Apply to acne scars or active breakouts for healing properties.

Brightening Lemon and Carrot Seed Roll-On

This brightening roll-on features the revitalizing effects of lemon essential oil and the nourishing properties of carrot seed oil. Lemon oil helps lighten dark spots and even skin tone, while carrot seed oil is rich in antioxidants and vitamins that support skin regeneration and repair. Together, they work to diminish the appearance of acne scars and promote a brighter, more radiant complexion.

What You Will Need:

- 6 drops Lemon essential oil
- 4 drops Carrot Seed essential oil
- 8 drops Tea Tree essential oil
- 2 tablespoons Grapeseed oil
- 10 ml glass roll-on bottle
- Small funnel (optional)
- Measuring spoons

What To Do:

1. Combine lemon, carrot seed, and tea tree oils using a funnel in the roll-on bottle.
2. Fill the remainder of the bottle with grapeseed oil.
3. Secure the rollerball top and cap, then shake to mix.
4. Use on dark spots or acne-prone areas to brighten and balance the skin.

Soothing Chamomile and Sandalwood Roll-On

This soothing roll-on blends the calming properties of chamomile essential oil with the grounding effects of sandalwood oil. Chamomile reduces redness and irritation, making it ideal for sensitive, acne-prone skin. Sandalwood oil provides deep relaxation while helping balance and clarify the skin. Together, they create a gentle treatment that soothes inflammation and supports a more even, clear complexion.

What You Will Need:

- 6 drops Roman Chamomile essential oil
- 5 drops Sandalwood essential oil
- 7 drops Lavender essential oil
- 2 tablespoons Sweet Almond oil
- 10 ml glass roll-on bottle
- Small funnel (optional)
- Measuring spoons

What To Do:

1. Using a funnel, add Roman chamomile, sandalwood, and lavender oil to the roll-on bottle.
2. Pour sweet almond oil into the bottle to fill the remaining space.
3. Attach the rollerball top and cap, then shake well.
4. Apply to inflamed or irritated areas of the skin for a soothing effect.

Blemish-Fighting Oregano and Tea Tree Roll-On

This powerful roll-on combines oregano essential oil's antibacterial properties with tea tree oil's purifying effects. Oregano oil is known for its strong antimicrobial action, making it highly effective against acne-causing bacteria. Tea tree oil complements this by helping to unclog pores and reduce the appearance of blemishes. Together, they create a potent treatment that targets and diminishes breakouts, leaving your skin clearer and healthier.

What You Will Need:

- 4 drops Oregano essential oil
- 8 drops Tea Tree essential oil
- 6 drops Lavender essential oil
- 2 tablespoons Jojoba oil
- 10 ml glass roll-on bottle
- Small funnel (optional)
- Measuring spoons

What To Do:

1. Using a funnel, add oregano, tea tree, and lavender oils to the roll-on bottle.
2. Fill the remainder of the bottle with jojoba oil.
3. Secure the rollerball top and cap, then shake to blend.
4. Apply sparingly to blemishes as a powerful spot treatment.

Anti-Redness Frankincense and Lavender Roll-On

This calming roll-on blend uses lavender essential oil's soothing properties with frankincense's anti-inflammatory benefits. Lavender helps to reduce skin irritation and redness, while frankincense promotes healing and evens skin tone. Together, they work to calm inflamed acne-prone areas, providing relief and supporting the skin's natural healing process.

What You Will Need:

- 7 drops Frankincense essential oil
- 6 drops Lavender essential oil
- 7 drops Helichrysum essential oil
- 2 tablespoons Rosehip Seed oil
- 10 ml glass roll-on bottle
- Small funnel (optional)
- Measuring spoons

What To Do:

1. Using a funnel, combine frankincense, lavender, and helichrysum oils in the roll-on bottle.
2. Add rosehip seed oil to fill the remainder of the bottle.
3. Attach the rollerball top and cap, then shake to combine.
4. Roll onto red, irritated areas to reduce inflammation and promote healing.

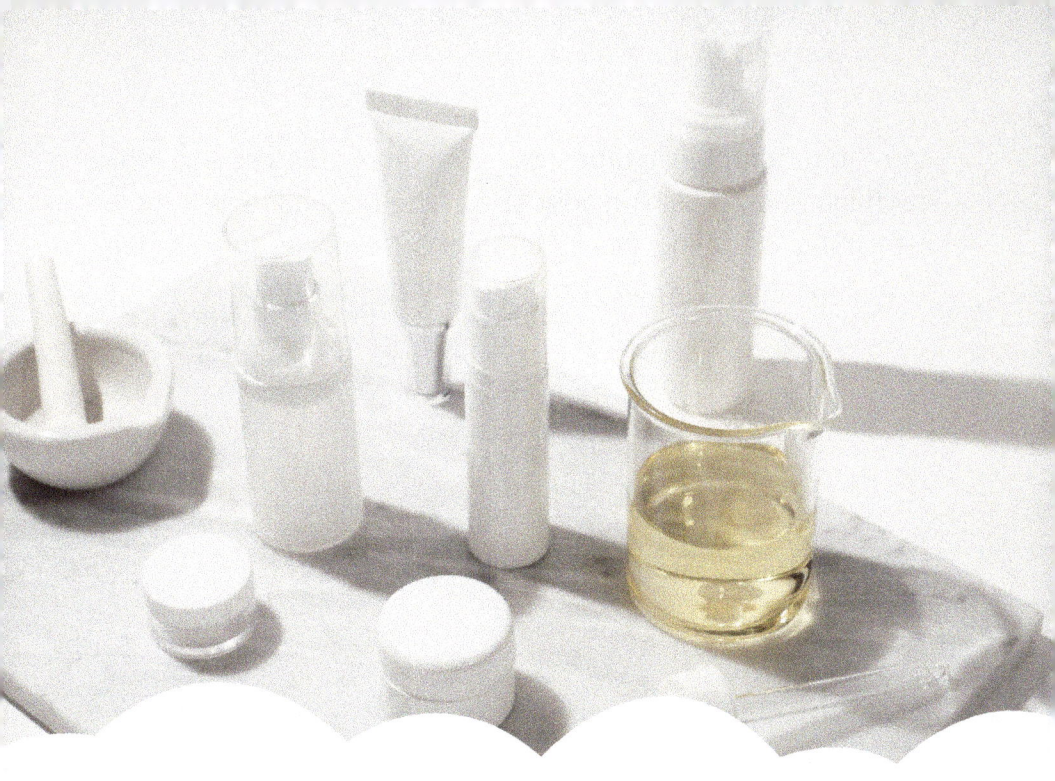

Chapter 16
Body Cleanser Recipes

Cleansers are the foundation of any effective skincare routine, especially when managing acne. They work to remove dirt, excess oil, makeup, and impurities that can clog pores and lead to breakouts. The right cleanser purifies the skin and prepares it to absorb the benefits of subsequent skincare products, such as toners, serums, and moisturizers. In this section, you'll find a variety of gentle yet powerful cleansers crafted with natural ingredients and essential oils. These recipes are designed to cater to different skin types, targeting acne at its source while soothing and nourishing your skin. Whether you're looking for a refreshing, clarifying, or hydrating cleanse, these formulations offer a tailored approach to clear, healthy-looking skin.

Gentle Tea Tree Cleanser

This gentle cleanser harnesses the antibacterial power of tea tree essential oil to effectively cleanse the skin without stripping it of its natural moisture, making it ideal for acne-prone skin.

What You Will Need:

- 1/4 cup Castile soap
- 1/4 cup Distilled water
- 10 drops Tea Tree essential oil
- 5 drops Lavender essential oil
- 1 tablespoon Aloe Vera gel
- Small mixing bowl
- Measuring cups and spoons
- Funnel (optional)
- 4 oz pump bottle or flip-top bottle

What To Do:

1. In a small mixing bowl, combine castile soap and distilled water.
2. Add tea tree, lavender, and aloe vera gel to the mixture.
3. Stir well to ensure all ingredients are thoroughly combined.
4. Using a funnel, pour the mixture into a 4 oz pump bottle or flip-top bottle.
5. Pump a small amount into your hands, gently massage onto the face, and rinse thoroughly with water.

Clarifying Lemon Cleanser

This cleanser combines the astringent properties of lemon essential oil to help clear away excess oil and impurities, leaving the skin feeling refreshed and clarified.

What You Will Need:

- 1/4 cup Unscented liquid soap
- 1/4 cup Distilled water
- 10 drops Lemon essential oil
- 5 drops Eucalyptus essential oil
- 1 tablespoon Honey
- Small mixing bowl
- Measuring cups and spoons
- Whisk or spoon for mixing
- Funnel (optional)
- 4 oz pump bottle or flip-top bottle

What To Do:

1. In a small mixing bowl, combine unscented liquid soap and distilled water.
2. Add lemon, eucalyptus, and honey, then whisk or stir until well-mixed.
3. Using a funnel, transfer the mixture into a 4 oz pump bottle or flip-top bottle.
4. Apply a small amount to damp skin, gently massage in circular motions, and rinse off with water.

Balancing Geranium Cleanser

This cleanser uses geranium and lavender essential oils to help balance the skin's oil production, making it ideal for maintaining a healthy complexion.

What You Will Need:

- 1/4 cup Castile soap
- 1/4 cup Rose Water
- 8 drops Geranium essential oil
- 5 drops Lavender essential oil
- 1 teaspoon Glycerin
- Small mixing bowl
- Measuring cups and spoons
- Funnel (optional)
- 4 oz pump bottle or flip-top bottle

What To Do:

1. In a small mixing bowl, combine castile soap and rose water.
2. Add geranium, lavender, and glycerin, stirring well to mix.
3. Using a funnel, pour the mixture into a 4 oz pump bottle or flip-top bottle.
4. Apply to damp skin, massage gently, and rinse off with warm water.

Revitalizing Peppermint Cleanser

This cleanser invigorates the skin with peppermint essential oil, leaving it feeling refreshed and revitalized while helping to control excess oil.

What You Will Need:

- 1/4 cup Unscented liquid soap
- 1/4 cup Distilled water
- 8 drops Peppermint essential oil
- 5 drops Tea Tree essential oil
- 1 teaspoon Vegetable glycerin
- Small mixing bowl
- Measuring cups and spoons
- Funnel (optional)
- 4 oz pump bottle or flip-top bottle

What To Do:

1. Combine unscented liquid soap and distilled water in a small mixing bowl.
2. Add peppermint, tea tree, and vegetable glycerin, stirring until well blended.
3. Use a funnel to pour the mixture into a 4 oz pump bottle or flip-top bottle.
4. To use, apply a small amount to the face, massage in circular motions, and rinse off.

Soothing Chamomile Cleanser

This cleanser gently soothes and calms the skin with chamomile essential oil, making it ideal for sensitive or irritated skin.

What You Will Need:

- 1/4 cup Castile soap
- 1/4 cup Chamomile Tea (cooled)
- 8 drops Roman Chamomile essential oil
- 5 drops Lavender essential oil
- 1 teaspoon Honey
- Small mixing bowl
- Measuring cups and spoons
- Funnel (optional)
- 4 oz pump bottle or flip-top bottle

What To Do:

1. Brew a small amount of chamomile tea and allow it to cool.
2. In a small mixing bowl, combine castile soap and cooled chamomile tea.
3. Add Roman chamomile, lavender, and honey, stirring well.
4. Pour the mixture into a 4 oz pump bottle or flip-top bottle using a funnel.
5. Apply to the face, massage gently, and rinse off with warm water.

Detoxifying Charcoal Cleanser

This cleanser deeply detoxifies the skin by drawing out impurities and excess oil with activated charcoal, helping to prevent breakouts and promote a clearer complexion.

What You Will Need:

- 1/4 cup Castile soap
- 1/4 cup Distilled water
- 1 teaspoon Activated Charcoal powder
- 10 drops Tea Tree essential oil
- 5 drops Lemon essential oil
- Small mixing bowl
- Measuring cups and spoons
- Whisk or spoon for mixing
- Funnel (optional)
- 4 oz pump bottle or flip-top bottle

What To Do:

1. In a small mixing bowl, combine castile soap and distilled water.
2. Add activated charcoal powder, tea tree, and lemon oil, whisking until smooth.
3. Using a funnel, pour the mixture into a 4 oz pump bottle or flip-top bottle.
4. Use a small amount to cleanse the face, focusing on areas with breakouts, then rinse thoroughly.

Calming Aloe and Lavender Cleanser

This cleanser soothes irritated skin with aloe vera and lavender's gentle, nourishing properties, making it ideal for sensitive or acne-prone skin.

What You Will Need:

- 1/4 cup Unscented liquid soap
- 1/4 cup Aloe Vera juice
- 8 drops Lavender essential oil
- 5 drops Frankincense essential oil
- 1 teaspoon Vegetable glycerin
- Small mixing bowl
- Measuring cups and spoons
- Funnel (optional)
- 4 oz pump bottle or flip-top bottle

What To Do:

1. Combine unscented liquid soap and aloe vera juice in a small mixing bowl.
2. Add lavender and frankincense oils and vegetable glycerin, stirring well.
3. Pour the mixture into a 4 oz pump bottle or flip-top bottle using a funnel.
4. Apply to damp skin, massage gently, and rinse with water.

Brightening Citrus Cleanser

This cleanser revitalizes and brightens the skin, harnessing the refreshing and clarifying properties of citrus essential oils to help reduce dullness and promote a glowing complexion.

What You Will Need:

- 1/4 cup Castile soap
- 1/4 cup Distilled water
- 8 drops Lemon essential oil
- 5 drops Grapefruit essential oil
- 1 teaspoon Honey
- Small mixing bowl
- Measuring cups and spoons
- Whisk or spoon for mixing
- Funnel (optional)
- 4 oz pump bottle or flip-top bottle

What To Do:

1. Combine castile soap and distilled water in a small mixing bowl.
2. Add lemon, grapefruit, and honey, whisking until smooth.
3. Use a funnel to pour the mixture into a 4 oz pump bottle or flip-top bottle.
4. To use, apply a small amount to the face, gently massage, and rinse off.

Exfoliating Oat and Lavender Cleanser

This cleanser combines the gentle exfoliating properties of oats with the soothing effects of lavender essential oil to remove dead skin cells, unclog pores, and calm irritation, leaving the skin refreshed and smooth.

What You Will Need:

- 1/4 cup Unscented liquid soap
- 1/4 cup Distilled water
- 1 tablespoon finely ground Oats
- 8 drops Lavender essential oil
- 5 drops Tea Tree essential oil
- Small mixing bowl
- Measuring cups and spoons
- Whisk or spoon for mixing
- Funnel (optional)
- 4 oz Pump bottle or flip-top bottle

What To Do:

1. In a small mixing bowl, combine unscented liquid soap and distilled water.
2. Add finely ground oats, lavender, and tea tree oils and whisk to combine.
3. Pour the mixture into a 4 oz pump bottle or flip-top bottle using a funnel.
4. Use as a gentle exfoliating cleanser, massaging onto the face and rinsing thoroughly.

Nourishing Honey and Almond Cleanser

This cleanser blends the moisturizing benefits of honey with the gentle exfoliation of almond milk, helping to nourish and soften the skin while effectively removing impurities.

What You Will Need:

- 1/4 cup Castile soap
- 1/4 cup Almond milk
- 8 drops Frankincense essential oil
- 5 drops Geranium essential oil
- 1 tablespoon Honey
- Small mixing bowl
- Measuring cups and spoons
- Whisk or spoon for mixing
- Funnel (optional)
- 4 oz pump bottle or flip-top bottle

What To Do:

1. Combine castile soap and almond milk in a small mixing bowl.
2. Add frankincense, geranium, and honey, whisking until thoroughly blended.
3. Transfer the mixture to a 4 oz pump bottle or flip-top bottle using a funnel.
4. Apply to damp skin, gently massage, and rinse off.

Hydrating Rose and Aloe Cleanser

This cleanser combines aloe vera's soothing properties with rose's hydrating benefits, providing gentle cleansing while replenishing moisture to the skin.

What You Will Need:

- 1/4 cup Unscented liquid soap
- 1/4 cup Rose Water
- 8 drops Rose essential oil
- 5 drops Lavender essential oil
- 1 tablespoon Aloe Vera gel
- Small mixing bowl
- Measuring cups and spoons
- Funnel (optional)
- 4 oz pump bottle or flip-top bottle

What To Do:

1. In a small mixing bowl, combine unscented liquid soap and rose water.
2. Add rose, lavender, and aloe vera gel, stirring well to blend.
3. Use a funnel to pour the mixture into a 4 oz pump bottle or flip-top bottle.
4. Apply to the face, massage gently, and rinse with warm water.

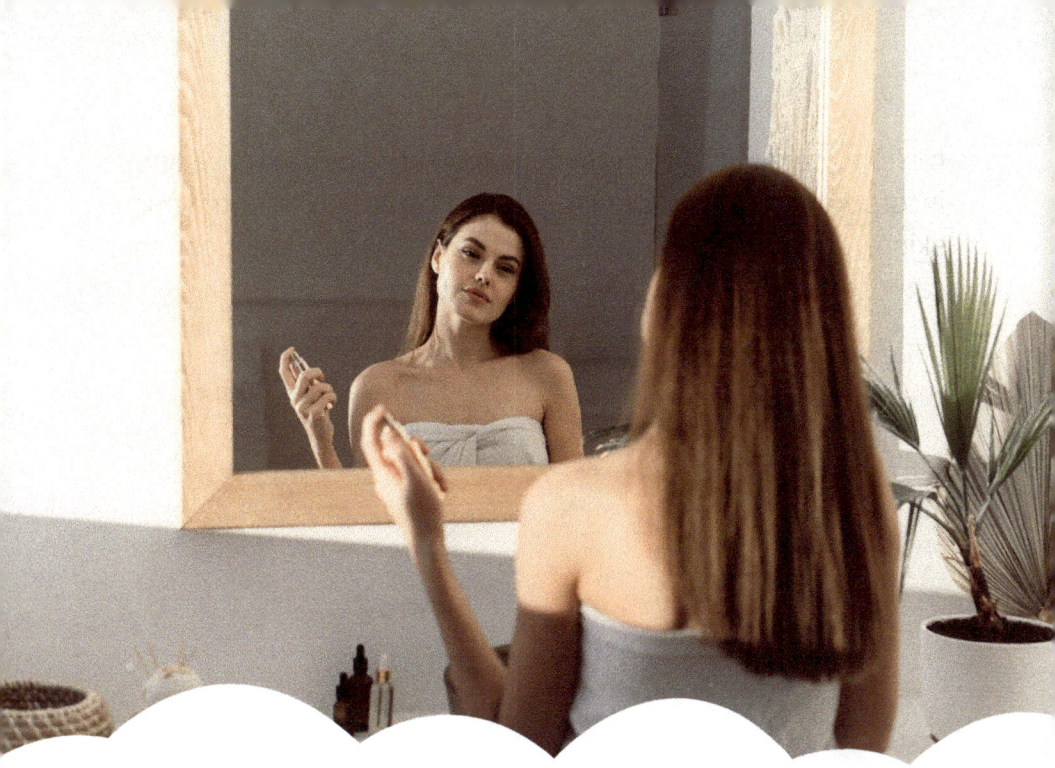

Chapter 17
Facial Mists and Spray Recipes

Facial sprays are a versatile and refreshing addition to any skincare routine, offering a quick and convenient way to address various skin concerns. Whether you're looking to combat acne, soothe inflammation, or simply refresh your complexion, these sprays can provide targeted relief and revitalization. This section will explore a selection of DIY facial spray recipes, each designed to harness the benefits of essential oils and natural ingredients. From acne-fighting mists to calming toners, these sprays are easy to make and incorporate into your daily regimen. Prepare to elevate your skincare routine with these effective, all-natural solutions that cater to different skin needs and preferences.

Acne-Fighting Facial Mist

This facial mist delivers a refreshing burst of hydration while targeting acne with powerful essential oils, helping to reduce breakouts and soothe irritated skin.

What You Will Need:

- 1/2 cup Distilled water
- 2 tablespoons Witch Hazel
- 10 drops Tea Tree essential oil
- 5 drops Peppermint essential oil
- Small mixing bowl
- Whisk or spoon for mixing
- 2 oz spray bottle
- Funnel (optional, for easy pouring)

What To Do:

1. Combine all ingredients in a small mixing bowl or directly in the spray bottle.
2. Whisk or stir well to ensure an even distribution of essential oils.
3. Pour the mixture into the spray bottle using a funnel if needed.
4. Shake well before each use.
5. Spritz onto the face after cleansing, avoiding the eyes.

Refreshing Antibacterial Spray

This antibacterial spray offers a quick and refreshing way to cleanse and protect the skin, using essential oils known for their ability to kill bacteria and prevent acne breakouts.

What You Will Need:

- 1/2 cup Distilled water
- 2 tablespoons Apple Cider Vinegar
- 10 drops Lavender essential oil
- 5 drops Eucalyptus essential oil
- Small mixing bowl
- Whisk or spoon for mixing
- 2 oz spray bottle
- Funnel (optional, for easy pouring)

What To Do:

1. Combine all ingredients in a small mixing bowl or directly in the spray bottle.
2. Whisk or stir well to mix the essential oils with the liquids.
3. Pour the mixture into the spray bottle using a funnel if needed.
4. Shake well before each use.
5. Use as a refreshing mist throughout the day to control bacteria and oil.

Calming Facial Toner Spray

This calming facial toner spray soothes irritated skin and reduces redness, helping to restore balance and promote a clearer complexion.

What You Will Need:

- 1/2 cup Rose Water
- 1/4 cup Distilled water
- 10 drops Roman Chamomile essential oil
- 5 drops Helichrysum essential oil
- Small mixing bowl
- Whisk or spoon for mixing
- 2 oz spray bottle
- Funnel (optional, for easy pouring)

What To Do:

1. Combine all ingredients in a small mixing bowl or directly in the spray bottle.
2. Whisk or stir well to blend the essential oils with the liquids.
3. Pour the mixture into the spray bottle using a funnel if needed.
4. Shake well before each use.
5. Spritz onto the face to soothe and balance the skin.

Purifying Detox Spray

This purifying detox spray helps cleanse the skin of impurities, leaving it refreshed and rejuvenated.

What You Will Need:

- 1/2 cup Distilled water
- 1/4 cup Aloe Vera juice
- 10 drops Lemon essential oil
- 5 drops Tea Tree essential oil
- 1 teaspoon Bentonite Clay (optional for added detoxification)
- Small mixing bowl
- Whisk or spoon for mixing
- 4 oz spray bottle
- Funnel (optional, for easy pouring)
- Small sieve (optional if using Bentonite Clay to ensure no lumps)

What To Do:

1. Combine distilled water, aloe vera juice, lemon, and tea tree oils in a small mixing bowl.
2. If using bentonite clay, add it to the mixture and whisk until fully dissolved.
3. Pour the mixture into the spray bottle using a funnel if needed.
4. Shake well before each use.
5. Spray onto the face, allowing it to dry naturally.

Aloe Vera and Rose Water Face Mist

This soothing face mist combines aloe vera's hydrating properties with rose water's calming effects to refresh and revitalize the skin.

What You Will Need:

- 2 tablespoons Aloe Vera gel
- 2 tablespoons Rose Water
- 1 tablespoon Distilled water
- 1 drop Lavender essential oil (optional)
- Small mixing bowl
- Whisk or spoon for mixing
- 2 oz spray bottle
- Funnel (optional, for easy pouring)

What To Do:

1. Combine the aloe vera gel and rose water in a small mixing bowl.
2. Stir in the distilled water until well combined.
3. If desired, add a drop of lavender essential oil.
4. Use a funnel to pour the mixture into the spray bottle.
5. Shake well before each use and spritz onto the face as needed.

Green Tea and Cucumber Face Mist

This refreshing face mist blends green tea's antioxidant benefits with cucumber's cooling effects to soothe and rejuvenate the skin.

What You Will Need:

- 1 cup Brewed Green Tea (cooled)
- 1/4 cup Cucumber juice
- 1 tablespoon Witch Hazel
- 1 drop Peppermint essential oil (optional)
- Small mixing bowl
- Fine strainer (for cucumber juice)
- 4 oz spray bottle
- Funnel (optional, for easy pouring)

What To Do:

1. Brew the green tea and let it cool to room temperature.
2. Combine the green tea, cucumber juice, and witch hazel in a mixing bowl.
3. If desired, add a drop of peppermint essential oil.
4. Use a funnel to pour the mixture into the spray bottle.
5. Shake well before each use and spritz onto the face for a refreshing boost.

Rose Water and Chamomile Face Mist

This gentle face mist combines rose water's calming properties with chamomile's soothing effects, providing a refreshing and hydrating boost for sensitive skin.

What You Will Need:

- 1/4 cup Rose Water
- 1/4 cup Chamomile Tea (cooled)
- 1 tablespoon Aloe Vera juice
- 1 drop of Roman Chamomile essential oil (optional)
- Small mixing bowl
- Whisk or spoon for mixing
- 2 oz spray bottle
- Funnel (optional, for easy pouring)

What To Do:

1. Brew chamomile tea and let it cool.
2. Mix rose water, chamomile tea, and aloe vera juice in a bowl.
3. If desired, add a drop of Roman chamomile essential oil.
4. Use a funnel to pour the mixture into the spray bottle.
5. Shake well before each use and spray onto the face to soothe and hydrate.

Green Tea and Mint Face Mist

This refreshing face mist blends the antioxidant power of green tea with the refreshing essence of mint, helping to rejuvenate and energize the skin.

What You Will Need:

- 1 cup Brewed Green Tea (cooled)
- 2 tablespoons Distilled water
- 1 tablespoon Aloe Vera gel
- 1 drop Spearmint essential oil (optional)
- Small mixing bowl
- Whisk or spoon for mixing
- 4 oz spray bottle
- Funnel (optional, for easy pouring)

What To Do:

1. Brew the green tea and let it cool.
2. Mix a bowl of green tea, distilled water, and aloe vera gel.
3. If desired, add a drop of spearmint essential oil.
4. Use a funnel to pour the mixture into the spray bottle.
5. Shake well before each use and mist onto your face for a refreshing pick-me-up.

Rose Water and Witch Hazel Face Mist

This soothing face mist combines rose water's hydrating properties with witch hazel's clarifying effects to calm and balance the skin while minimizing excess oil and refining pores.

What You Will Need:

- 1/4 cup Rose Water
- 1/4 cup Witch Hazel
- 1/4 cup Distilled water
- 1 drop Frankincense essential oil (optional)
- Small mixing bowl
- Whisk or spoon for mixing
- 2 oz spray bottle
- Funnel (optional, for easy pouring)

What To Do:

1. Combine rose water, witch hazel, and distilled water in a mixing bowl.
2. If desired, add a drop of frankincense essential oil.
3. Use a funnel to pour the mixture into the spray bottle.
4. Shake well before each use and spritz onto the face to tone and hydrate.

Aloe Vera and Green Tea Face Mist

This revitalizing face mist merges the soothing benefits of aloe vera with the antioxidant power of green tea, offering a refreshing boost that calms irritation and helps protect the skin from environmental stressors.

What You Will Need:

- 1/2 cup Brewed Green Tea (cooled)
- 1/4 cup Aloe Vera juice
- 1/4 cup Distilled water
- 1 drop Tea Tree essential oil (optional)
- Small mixing bowl
- Whisk or spoon for mixing
- 4 oz spray bottle
- Funnel (optional, for easy pouring)

What To Do:

1. Brew green tea and let it cool.
2. Combine green tea, aloe vera juice, and distilled water in a bowl.
3. If desired, add a drop of tea tree essential oil.
4. Use a funnel to pour the mixture into the spray bottle.
5. Shake well before each use and spray onto the face to calm and refresh.

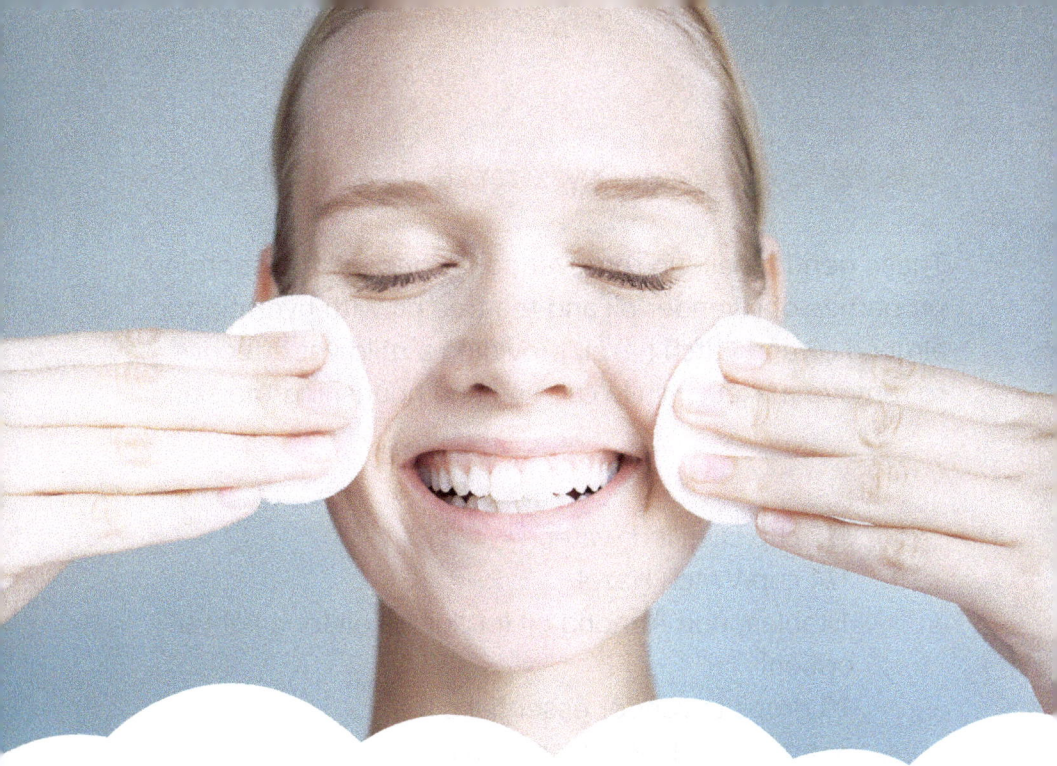

Chapter 18
Makeup Remover Pads

Makeup remover pads infused with essential oils can gently and effectively cleanse the skin while addressing acne and other skin concerns. These makeup remover pad recipes use essential oils and natural ingredients to clean the skin and address acne, inflammation, and other problems. Adjust the essential oil blends based on personal preferences and skin sensitivity. Here are a few recipes for makeup remover pads that incorporate essential oils.

Gentle Makeup Remover Pads

These gentle makeup remover pads combine the soothing properties of lavender oil and tea tree oil with hydrating almond oil and witch hazel, providing a mild yet effective way to remove makeup while calming and nourishing the skin.

What You Will Need:

- 1/2 cup Distilled water
- 1/4 cup Witch Hazel
- 1 tablespoon Almond oil (or Jojoba oil for a lighter option)
- 10 drops Lavender essential oil
- 5 drops Tea Tree essential oil
- 1-2 teaspoons Aloe Vera gel
- Mixing bowl
- Measuring cups and spoons
- Spoon or whisk
- Reusable cotton pads or pre-cut cotton rounds
- Airtight glass jar or container

What To Do:

1. Combine the distilled water, witch hazel, and almond oil (or jojoba oil) in a mixing bowl.
2. Stir in the lavender, tea tree, and aloe vera gel until well combined.
3. Place the reusable cotton pads or pre-cut cotton rounds into the mixture, ensuring they are fully saturated.
4. Transfer the soaked pads into an airtight glass jar or container.
5. Use a pad to remove makeup, then gently rinse.

Refreshing Citrus Makeup Remover Pads

These refreshing citrus makeup remover pads utilize the zesty benefits of lemon, grapefruit, and coconut oils, creating a revitalizing formula that removes makeup and brightens and refreshes the skin.

What You Will Need:

- 1/2 cup Distilled water
- 1/4 cup Coconut oil
- 10 drops Lemon essential oil
- 5 drops Grapefruit essential oil
- 1 tablespoon Apple Cider Vinegar
- Mixing bowl
- Measuring cups and spoons
- Spoon or whisk
- Reusable cotton pads or pre-cut cotton rounds
- Airtight glass jar or container

What To Do:

1. Combine distilled water, coconut oil, and apple cider vinegar in a mixing bowl.
2. Add lemon and grapefruit oils to the bowl and mix until the coconut oil is fully incorporated.
3. Place the reusable cotton pads or pre-cut cotton rounds into the mixture, ensuring they are evenly saturated.
4. Store the soaked pads in an airtight glass jar or container.
5. Use to remove makeup and impurities gently.

Calming Rose Water Makeup Remover Pads

These calming rose water makeup remover pads combine the soothing properties of rose water and chamomile with gentle jojoba oil, offering a delicate formula that removes makeup while calming and hydrating sensitive skin.

What You Will Need:

- 1/2 cup Rose Water
- 1/4 cup Witch Hazel
- 1 tablespoon Jojoba oil
- 5 drops Roman Chamomile essential oil
- 5 drops Geranium essential oil
- 1 tablespoon Aloe Vera gel
- Mixing bowl
- Measuring cups and spoons
- Spoon or whisk
- Reusable cotton pads or pre-cut cotton rounds
- Airtight glass jar or container

What To Do:

1. Combine the rose water, witch hazel, jojoba oil, and aloe vera gel in a mixing bowl.
2. Add the Roman chamomile and geranium oils, then stir well.
3. Place the reusable cotton pads or pre-cut cotton rounds into the solution, ensuring they are thoroughly soaked.
4. Store the soaked pads in a sealed glass jar or container.
5. Gently use a pad to remove makeup and soothe the skin.

Hydrating Makeup Remover Pads

These hydrating makeup remover pads feature a nourishing blend of fractionated coconut oil and frankincense essential oil, designed to effectively remove makeup while providing deep hydration and soothing benefits for a refreshed complexion.

What You Will Need:

- 1/2 cup Distilled water
- 1/4 cup Fractionated Coconut oil
- 10 drops Frankincense essential oil
- 5 drops Lavender essential oil
- 1 tablespoon Aloe Vera juice
- Mixing bowl
- Measuring cups and spoons
- Spoon or whisk
- Reusable cotton pads or pre-cut cotton rounds
- Airtight glass jar or container

What To Do:

1. Combine the distilled water, fractionated coconut oil, and aloe vera juice in a mixing bowl.
2. Add the frankincense and lavender oils, then mix thoroughly until well blended.
3. Saturate the reusable cotton pads or pre-cut cotton rounds with the solution.
4. Place the soaked pads in an airtight glass jar or container.
5. Use a pad to remove makeup while hydrating the skin.

Detoxifying Green Tea Makeup Remover Pads

Infused with the detoxifying power of green tea and the clarifying properties of tea tree oil, these makeup remover pads help to cleanse and refresh the skin, removing impurities while providing a purifying boost.

What You Will Need:

- 1/2 cup Brewed Green Tea (cooled)
- 1/4 cup Witch Hazel
- 1 tablespoon Almond oil
- 10 drops Tea Tree essential oil
- 5 drops Lemon essential oil
- Mixing bowl
- Measuring cups and spoons
- Spoon or whisk
- Reusable cotton pads or pre-cut cotton rounds
- Airtight glass jar or container

What To Do:

1. Brew the green tea and allow it to cool completely.
2. Combine the cooled green tea, witch hazel, and almond oil in a mixing bowl.
3. Add tea tree and lemon essential oils, then stir to combine.
4. Place the reusable cotton pads or pre-cut cotton rounds into the mixture, ensuring they are fully saturated.
5. Store the soaked pads in an airtight glass jar or container.
6. Use a pad to remove makeup and refresh the skin.

Soothing Aloe and Cucumber Makeup Remover Pads

Designed to soothe and hydrate, these makeup remover pads combine aloe vera and cucumber to calm irritated skin and gently remove makeup, leaving your complexion refreshed and revitalized.

What You Will Need:

- 1/2 cup Distilled water
- 1/4 cup Aloe Vera gel
- 2 tablespoons Cucumber juice (freshly extracted)
- 10 drops Chamomile essential oil
- 5 drops Lavender essential oil
- Mixing bowl
- Measuring cups and spoons
- Spoon or whisk
- Reusable cotton pads or pre-cut cotton rounds
- Airtight glass jar or container

What To Do:

1. Combine distilled water, aloe vera gel, and cucumber juice in a mixing bowl.
2. Add chamomile and lavender oils, then stir until well combined.
3. Place the reusable cotton pads or pre-cut cotton rounds into the mixture, ensuring they are fully saturated.
4. Store the soaked pads in an airtight glass jar or container.
5. Use a pad to remove makeup and soothe the skin gently.

Anti-Inflammatory Calendula Makeup Remover Pads

These anti-inflammatory makeup remover pads feature calendula to soothe and calm irritated skin while effectively removing makeup, making them ideal for sensitive or inflamed skin.

What You Will Need:

- 1/2 cup Calendula-infused water (steep dried calendula flowers in hot water and cool)
- 1/4 cup Witch Hazel
- 1 tablespoon Jojoba oil
- 10 drops Frankincense essential oil
- 5 drops Tea Tree essential oil
- Mixing bowl
- Measuring cups and spoons
- Spoon or whisk
- Reusable cotton pads or pre-cut cotton rounds
- Airtight glass jar or container

What To Do:

1. Prepare calendula-infused water and allow it to cool.
2. Combine the calendula-infused water, witch hazel, and jojoba oil in a mixing bowl.
3. Add frankincense and tea tree oils, then stir to blend the ingredients.
4. Saturate the reusable cotton pads or pre-cut cotton rounds with the mixture.
5. Place the soaked pads in an airtight glass jar or container.
6. Use a pad to remove makeup while calming inflammation.

Brightening Neroli Makeup Remover Pads

These brightening makeup remover pads use neroli to enhance radiance and even out skin tone while gently cleansing away makeup and impurities for a luminous complexion.

What You Will Need:

- 1/2 cup Neroli floral water
- 1/4 cup Sweet Almond oil
- 10 drops Sweet Orange essential oil
- 5 drops Neroli essential oil
- Mixing bowl
- Measuring cups and spoons
- Spoon or whisk
- Reusable cotton pads or pre-cut cotton rounds
- Airtight glass jar or container

What To Do:

1. In a mixing bowl, combine neroli floral water and sweet almond oil.
2. Add sweet orange and neroli oils, then mix until well combined.
3. Soak the reusable cotton pads or pre-cut cotton rounds in the mixture.
4. Store the soaked pads in an airtight glass jar or container.
5. Use to remove makeup and brighten the complexion gently.

Clarifying Mint and Lemon Makeup Remover Pads

These clarifying makeup remover pads combine the refreshing properties of mint with the brightening effects of lemon, helping to clear away makeup while invigorating and balancing the skin.

What You Will Need:

- 1/2 cup Distilled water
- 1/4 cup Aloe Vera juice
- 10 drops Peppermint essential oil
- 5 drops Lemon essential oil
- 1 teaspoon Vegetable glycerin (optional for added moisture)
- Mixing bowl
- Measuring cups and spoons
- Spoon or whisk
- Reusable cotton pads or pre-cut cotton rounds
- Airtight glass jar or container

What To Do:

1. In a mixing bowl, combine distilled water and aloe vera juice.
2. Add peppermint, lemon, and vegetable glycerin (if used), then stir well.
3. Place the reusable cotton pads or pre-cut cotton rounds into the mixture, ensuring they are fully saturated.
4. Store the soaked pads in an airtight glass jar or container.
5. Use to remove makeup while refreshing and clarifying the skin.

Deep Cleansing Charcoal Makeup Remover Pads

These deep-cleansing makeup remover pads feature charcoal to draw out impurities and toxins, ensuring a thorough cleanse while removing makeup and leaving the skin fresh and revitalized.

What You Will Need:

- 1/2 cup Distilled water
- 1/4 cup Witch Hazel
- 1 tablespoon Activated Charcoal powder
- 10 drops Tea Tree essential oil
- 5 drops Rosemary essential oil
- Mixing bowl
- Measuring cups and spoons
- Spoon or whisk
- Reusable cotton pads or pre-cut cotton rounds
- Airtight glass jar or container

What To Do:

1. In a mixing bowl, combine distilled water and witch hazel.
2. Add the activated charcoal powder, tea tree, and rosemary oils, stirring until the charcoal is fully dissolved.
3. Saturate the reusable cotton pads or pre-cut cotton rounds with the mixture.
4. Store the soaked pads in an airtight glass jar or container.
5. Use to remove makeup while deeply cleansing and detoxifying the skin.

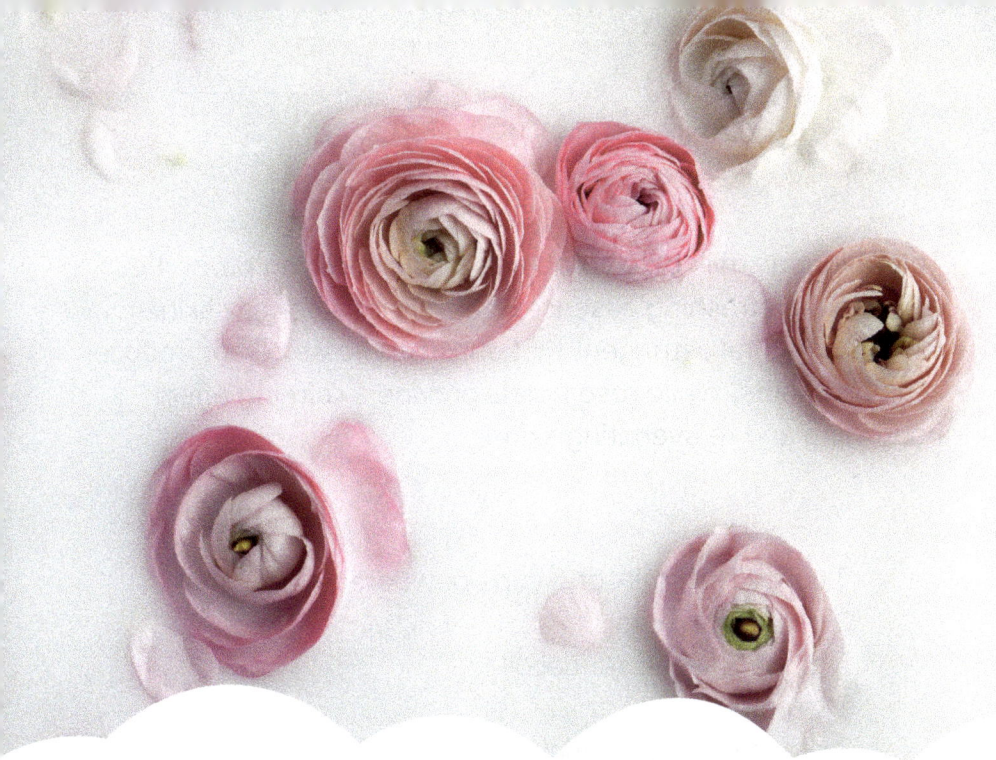

Chapter 19
Milk Baths

Milk baths offer a luxurious and soothing way to address acne while providing numerous skin benefits. Combining essential oils with milk, whether fresh or powdered, creates a nourishing and hydrating experience for the skin. The gentle exfoliating properties of milk, enriched with essential oils, can help soothe inflammation, balance oil production, and promote a clearer complexion. In this section, you'll find recipes for milk baths that blend the calming effects of essential oils with the skin-loving properties of milk, offering a refreshing approach to managing acne and enhancing your skincare routine.

Rose and Lime Milk Bath

This luxurious milk bath combines rose's soothing properties with lime's refreshing essence, which is ideal for oily skin. Lime is a natural astringent that absorbs excess oil and reduces acne breakouts, while rose petals provide a calming effect, nourishing and rejuvenating skin.

What You Will Need:

- 3 cups Fresh milk or 2 cups powdered milk
- 2 cups Rose petals
- 5 drops Rose essential oil
- 3 Limes
- 3 drops Lime essential oil
- Medium bowl
- Knife for slicing limes
- Measuring cups

What To Do:

1. Slice 2 limes and squeeze the juice into a medium bowl. Add the lime essential oil to the bowl.
2. Mix in 1 cup of rose petals and either fresh or powdered milk. Stir well to combine.
3. Pour the mixture into running bathwater.
4. Slice the third lime and add it to the bath with the remaining cup of rose petals to float on top.

Lavender and Oatmeal Milk Bath

This soothing milk bath combines lavender and oatmeal to calm and nourish your skin gently. Lavender's relaxing scent helps reduce stress while its calming properties ease skin irritation, and oatmeal offers gentle exfoliation and hydration, perfect for sensitive or dry skin.

What You Will Need:

- 2 cups Powdered milk
- 1/2 cup finely ground Oatmeal
- 10 drops Lavender essential oil
- Mixing bowl
- Whisk or spoon for mixing
- Airtight jar or container for storage

What To Do:

1. In a mixing bowl, combine powdered milk and ground oatmeal.
2. Add lavender oil and mix thoroughly until well combined.
3. Pour the mixture into warm bathwater, stirring to dissolve.
4. Soak in the bath for 20-30 minutes, allowing the ingredients to soothe and cleanse the skin.

Tea Tree and Epsom Salt Milk Bath

This invigorating milk bath combines tea tree oil with epsom salt to help cleanse and rejuvenate the skin. Tea tree oil's natural antiseptic properties combat acne and inflammation, while epsom salt soothes and relaxes tired muscles, making this bath ideal for a refreshing and therapeutic experience.

What You Will Need:

- 2 cups Powdered milk
- 1 cup Epsom salt
- 10 drops Tea Tree essential oil
- Mixing bowl
- Whisk or spoon for mixing
- Airtight jar or container for storage

What To Do:

1. In a mixing bowl, combine powdered milk and epsom salt.
2. Add tea tree oil and mix well until thoroughly blended.
3. Pour the mixture into warm bathwater, stirring to dissolve.
4. Soak in the bath for 20-30 minutes to help detoxify and treat acne-prone skin.

Chamomile and Honey Milk Bath

This soothing milk bath combines chamomile and honey to provide calming and moisturizing benefits. Chamomile's anti-inflammatory properties help to soothe irritated skin, while honey adds a layer of hydration, leaving the skin feeling soft and nourished.

What You Will Need:

- 2 cups Fresh milk or powdered milk
- 2 tablespoons Honey
- 10 drops Chamomile essential oil
- Mixing bowl
- Whisk or spoon for mixing
- Airtight jar or container for storage

What To Do:

1. In a mixing bowl, combine fresh or powdered milk with honey.
2. Add chamomile oil and mix thoroughly until well blended.
3. Pour the mixture into warm bathwater, stirring to dissolve.
4. Soak in the bath for 20-30 minutes, allowing the ingredients to calm and nourish the skin.

Rosemary and Sea Salt Milk Bath

This rejuvenating milk bath combines rosemary and sea salt to provide a refreshing and invigorating experience. Rosemary's stimulating properties help to energize and promote circulation, while sea salt helps to exfoliate and detoxify the skin, leaving it feeling refreshed and revitalized.

What You Will Need:

- 2 cups Powdered milk
- 1 cup Sea Salt
- 10 drops Rosemary essential oil
- Mixing bowl
- Whisk or spoon for mixing
- Airtight jar or container for storage

What To Do:

1. In a mixing bowl, combine powdered milk and sea salt.
2. Add rosemary oil and mix well until thoroughly combined.
3. Pour the mixture into warm bathwater, stirring to dissolve.
4. Soak in the bath for 20-30 minutes to help cleanse and rejuvenate acne-prone skin.

Peppermint and Green Tea Milk Bath

This invigorating milk bath blends peppermint and green tea to provide a refreshing and revitalizing experience. Peppermint's cooling effect soothes and rejuvenates the skin, while green tea's antioxidants help to combat free radicals and promote a healthy glow.

What You Will Need:

- 2 cups Powdered milk
- 1/2 cup Green Tea (brewed and cooled)
- 10 drops Peppermint essential oil
- Mixing bowl
- Whisk or spoon for mixing
- Airtight jar or container for storage

What To Do:

1. In a mixing bowl, combine powdered milk with brewed green tea.
2. Add peppermint oil and mix until well blended.
3. Pour the mixture into warm bathwater, stirring to dissolve.
4. Soak in the bath for 20-30 minutes, allowing the ingredients to refresh and soothe the skin.

Lemongrass and Coconut Milk Bath

This rejuvenating milk bath combines lemongrass and coconut milk to create a refreshing and hydrating soak. Lemongrass helps to invigorate and uplift the senses, while coconut milk nourishes and moisturizes the skin, leaving it feeling soft and revitalized.

What You Will Need:

- 2 cups Powdered coconut milk
- 1 cup Baking soda
- 10 drops Lemongrass essential oil
- Mixing bowl
- Whisk or spoon for mixing
- Airtight jar or container for storage

What To Do:

1. In a mixing bowl, combine powdered coconut milk and baking soda.
2. Add lemongrass oil and mix well until thoroughly combined.
3. Pour the mixture into warm bathwater, stirring to dissolve.
4. Soak in the bath for 20-30 minutes to cleanse and balance oily, acne-prone skin.

Frankincense and Almond Milk Bath

This luxurious milk bath blends the warm, resinous notes of frankincense with the nourishing properties of almond milk. Frankincense offers a soothing, grounding effect, while almond milk deeply hydrates and softens the skin, creating a calming and rejuvenating bath experience.

What You Will Need:

- 2 cups Powdered almond milk
- 1/2 cup Epsom salt
- 10 drops Frankincense essential oil
- Mixing bowl
- Whisk or spoon for mixing
- Airtight jar or container for storage

What To Do:

1. In a mixing bowl, combine powdered almond milk and epsom salt.
2. Add frankincense oil and mix until well blended.
3. Pour the mixture into warm bathwater, stirring to dissolve.
4. Soak in the bath for 20-30 minutes, allowing the ingredients to nourish and soothe the skin.

Geranium and Rose Milk Bath

This soothing milk bath combines geranium's floral elegance with the rose's delicate fragrance, offering a calming and uplifting experience. Geranium helps balance and tone the skin, while rose milk nourishes and hydrates, leaving your skin feeling soft and refreshed.

What You Will Need:

- 2 cups Powdered milk
- 1/2 cup Dried rose petals
- 10 drops Geranium essential oil
- Mixing bowl
- Whisk or spoon for mixing
- Airtight jar or container for storage

What To Do:

1. In a mixing bowl, combine powdered milk with dried rose petals.
2. Add geranium oil and mix thoroughly.
3. Pour the mixture into warm bathwater, stirring to dissolve.
4. Soak in the bath for 20-30 minutes to help balance and rejuvenate the skin.

Orange and Calendula Milk Bath

This rejuvenating milk bath blends the bright, uplifting scent of orange with the soothing properties of calendula. Orange helps to invigorate and refresh the skin, while calendula provides gentle, calming, and healing effects, making this bath ideal for a revitalizing and comforting soak.

What You Will Need:

- 2 cups Powdered milk
- 1/2 cup Dried calendula petals
- 10 drops Orange essential oil
- Mixing bowl
- Whisk or spoon for mixing
- Airtight jar or container for storage

What To Do:

1. In a mixing bowl, combine powdered milk with dried calendula petals.
2. Add orange oil and mix well until thoroughly combined.
3. Pour the mixture into warm bathwater, stirring to dissolve.
4. Soak in the bath for 20-30 minutes to brighten and tone acne-prone skin.

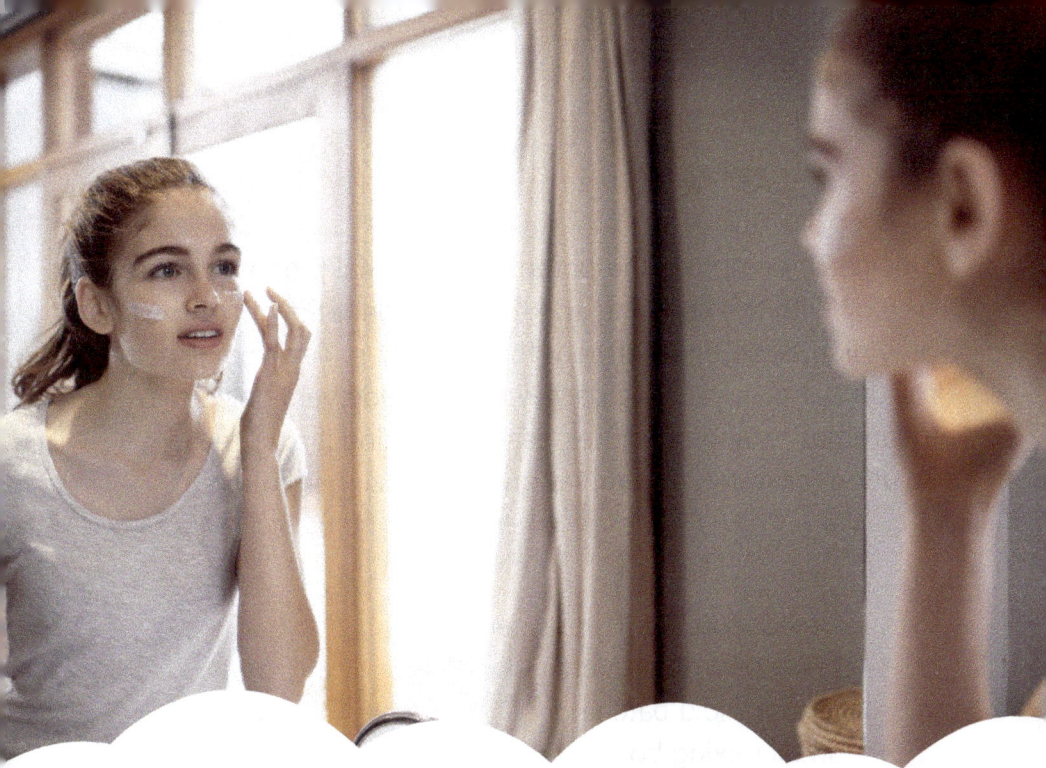

Chapter 20
Acne Patches

Acne patches are an effective and convenient way to target individual blemishes, delivering potent ingredients directly where needed most. These small, stick-on treatments address breakouts without disturbing the surrounding skin. Sealing the blemish creates a protective barrier that prevents further irritation and promotes faster healing. Essential oils can be incorporated into acne patches to enhance their therapeutic effects, offering antibacterial, anti-inflammatory, and soothing benefits.

Tea Tree and Aloe Vera Patch

This patch combines the potent antibacterial properties of tea tree oil with the soothing and hydrating benefits of aloe vera, providing targeted treatment for blemishes. Tea tree oil helps to combat acne-causing bacteria, while aloe vera helps calm inflammation and promotes healing, making it an effective solution for reducing pimples and minimizing irritation.

What You Will Need:

- 1 teaspoon Tea Tree essential oil
- 1 teaspoon Aloe Vera gel
- Hydrocolloid patches
- Small mixing bowl
- Clean spatula or spoon
- Airtight container for storing unused patches

What To Do:

1. Mix tea tree oil and aloe vera gel in a small bowl until well combined.
2. Dab a small amount onto each hydrocolloid patch.
3. Apply the patch to clean dry skin directly on the blemish.
4. Store unused patches in an airtight container.

Lavender and Witch Hazel Patch

This patch pairs calming lavender oil with the astringent properties of witch hazel to address acne-prone skin. Lavender oil helps to soothe and reduce inflammation, while witch hazel tightens pores and helps control excess oil. Together, they provide a balanced approach to calming irritated skin and promoting a clearer complexion.

What You Will Need:

- 1 teaspoon Lavender essential oil
- 1 teaspoon Witch Hazel
- Hydrocolloid patches
- Small mixing bowl
- Clean dropper
- Airtight container for storage

What To Do:

1. Combine lavender oil and witch hazel in a small bowl.
2. Use a dropper to apply a small amount to each hydrocolloid patch.
3. Apply the patch to the affected area and leave it on overnight.
4. Store the remaining patches in an airtight container.

Frankincense and Chamomile Patch

This soothing patch combines the calming properties of frankincense and chamomile to target blemishes and promote healing. Frankincense helps to reduce inflammation and diminish the appearance of scars, while chamomile provides gentle relief from irritation and redness. It is ideal for those looking to alleviate discomfort and support skin recovery.

What You Will Need:

- 1 teaspoon Frankincense essential oil
- 1 teaspoon Chamomile hydrosol
- Hydrocolloid patches
- Small mixing bowl
- Cotton swabs
- Airtight container for storage

What To Do:

1. Mix frankincense oil and chamomile hydrosol in a bowl.
2. Use a cotton swab to apply the mixture to each patch.
3. Place the patch on the blemish and leave it on for several hours.
4. Store the remaining patches in an airtight container.

Clary Sage and Rose Water Patch

The Clary Sage and Rose Water Patch combines the balancing and calming effects of clary sage with the soothing properties of rose water. This patch helps to regulate oil production and reduce redness, promoting a clearer and more balanced complexion. It is ideal for sensitive or acne-prone skin and supports healing while calming irritation and inflammation.

What You Will Need:

- 1 teaspoon Clary Sage essential oil
- 1 teaspoon Rose Water
- Hydrocolloid patches
- Small mixing bowl
- Clean dropper
- Airtight container for storage

What To Do:

1. Combine clary sage oil and rose water in a bowl.
2. Use a clean dropper to apply the mixture to the patches.
3. Adhere the patch to the acne spot and leave it on overnight.
4. Store unused patches in an airtight container.

Lemon and Honey Patch

The lemon and honey patch blends the clarifying properties of lemon with the moisturizing benefits of honey. This patch helps brighten and clarify the skin while providing gentle hydration, effectively reducing blemishes and promoting a more even skin tone.

What You Will Need:

- 1 teaspoon Lemon essential oil
- 1 teaspoon Honey
- Hydrocolloid patches
- Small mixing bowl
- Clean dropper
- Airtight container for storage

What To Do:

1. Mix lemon oil and honey in a bowl until well combined.
2. Apply a small amount to each hydrocolloid patch using a dropper.
3. Place the patch on the affected area and leave it on overnight.
4. Store the remaining patches in an airtight container.

Peppermint and Green Tea Patch

The Peppermint and Green Tea Patch combines the soothing and cooling effects of peppermint with the antioxidant-rich properties of green tea. This patch helps to calm irritated skin, reduce redness, and combat acne, offering a refreshing treatment that promotes a clearer and more balanced complexion.

What You Will Need:

- 1 teaspoon Peppermint essential oil
- 1 teaspoon Brewed Green Tea (cooled)
- Hydrocolloid patches
- Small mixing bowl
- Cotton swabs
- Airtight container for storage

What To Do:

1. Mix peppermint oil and cooled green tea in a bowl.
2. Use a cotton swab to apply the mixture to each patch.
3. Adhere the patch to the blemish and leave it on for several hours.
4. Store the remaining patches in an airtight container.

Geranium and Apple Cider Vinegar Patch

The Geranium and Apple Cider Vinegar Patch combines the balancing properties of geranium with the clarifying and pH-regulating effects of apple cider vinegar. This patch helps to reduce acne, balance oily skin, and refine pores, providing a gentle yet effective treatment for clearer, more even skin.

What You Will Need:

- 1 teaspoon Geranium essential oil
- 1 teaspoon Apple Cider Vinegar
- Hydrocolloid patches
- Small mixing bowl
- Clean dropper
- Airtight container for storage

What To Do:

1. Combine geranium oil and apple cider vinegar in a bowl.
2. Use a dropper to apply a small amount to each hydrocolloid patch.
3. Place the patch on the blemish and leave it on overnight.
4. Store the remaining patches in an airtight container.

Eucalyptus and Aloe Vera Patch

The Eucalyptus and Aloe Vera Patch utilizes eucalyptus' antimicrobial and soothing properties alongside aloe vera's calming and hydrating benefits. This combination helps to alleviate inflammation, reduce redness, and promote healing, making it ideal for treating irritated and blemish-prone skin.

What You Will Need:

- 1 teaspoon Eucalyptus essential oil
- 1 teaspoon Aloe Vera gel
- Hydrocolloid patches
- Small mixing bowl
- Clean dropper
- Airtight container for storage

What To Do:

1. Mix eucalyptus oil and aloe vera gel in a bowl until well combined.
2. Apply a small amount to each hydrocolloid patch.
3. Place the patch on the affected area and leave it on overnight.
4. Store the remaining patches in an airtight container.

Tea Tree and Jojoba Oil Patch

The Tea Tree and Jojoba Oil Patch combines the antiseptic and acne-fighting properties of tea tree oil with the moisturizing and balancing benefits of jojoba oil. This patch helps to target blemishes while maintaining skin hydration, reducing dryness, and preventing irritation.

What You Will Need:

- 1 teaspoon Tea Tree essential oil
- 1 teaspoon Jojoba oil
- Hydrocolloid patches
- Small mixing bowl
- Clean dropper
- Airtight container for storage

What To Do:

1. Combine tea tree oil and jojoba oil in a bowl.
2. Use a clean dropper to apply the mixture to the patches.
3. Adhere the patch to the acne spot and leave it on overnight.
4. Store unused patches in an airtight container.

Rosemary and Witch Hazel Patch

The Rosemary and Witch Hazel Patch harnesses the purifying and astringent qualities of rosemary and witch hazel to help reduce inflammation and tighten pores, providing a soothing and clarifying treatment for acne-prone skin.

What You Will Need:

- 1 teaspoon Rosemary essential oil
- 1 teaspoon Witch Hazel
- Hydrocolloid patches
- Small mixing bowl
- Clean dropper
- Airtight container for storage

What To Do:

1. Combine rosemary oil and witch hazel in a bowl.
2. Use a dropper to apply a small amount to each hydrocolloid patch.
3. Place the patch on the blemish and leave it on overnight.
4. Store the remaining patches in an airtight container.

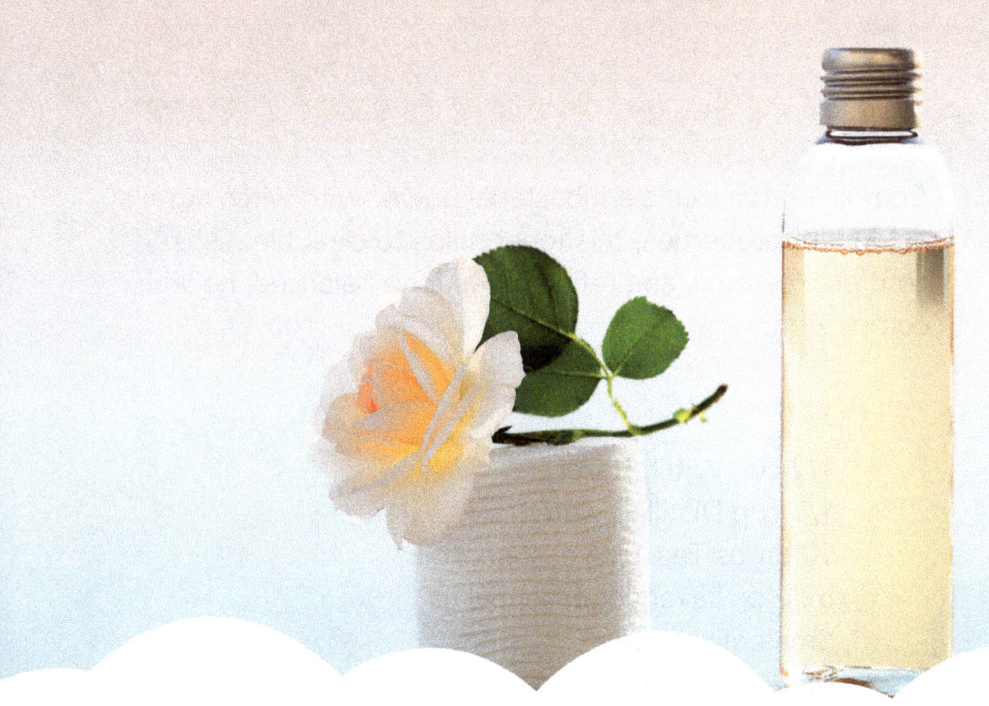

Chapter 21
Toners for Acne

Toners are crucial in any skincare routine, particularly for acne-prone skin. They help to balance the skin's pH, remove residual impurities after cleansing, and prepare the skin for further treatments. For those with acne, toners can be particularly beneficial in reducing excess oil, tightening pores, and soothing inflammation. When infused with essential oils, toners can offer additional antibacterial, anti-inflammatory, and skin-healing properties, effectively combating acne.

Tea Tree and Witch Hazel Toner

Combining tea tree's antibacterial power with witch hazel's astringent properties, this toner helps to clear blemishes, control excess oil, and refine pores for a balanced, healthier complexion.

What You Will Need:

- 1/2 cup Witch Hazel
- 1/2 cup Distilled water
- 10 drops Tea Tree essential oil
- 5 drops Lavender essential oil
- Small mixing bowl
- Measuring cups
- Funnel
- Glass or plastic spray bottle (4 oz.)

What To Do:

1. In a mixing bowl, combine witch hazel and distilled water.
2. Add tea tree and lavender essential oils, stirring well.
3. Use a funnel to pour the mixture into the spray bottle.
4. Shake well before each use, and apply with a cotton pad after cleansing.

Rose Water and Aloe Toner

This soothing toner blends rose water's hydrating benefits with aloe's calming properties, helping to refresh and balance the skin while reducing redness and irritation.

What You Will Need:

- 1/2 cup Rose Water
- 1/4 cup Aloe Vera juice
- 10 drops Geranium essential oil
- 5 drops Frankincense essential oil
- Small mixing bowl
- Measuring cups
- Funnel
- Glass bottle (4 oz.)

What To Do:

1. Combine rose water and aloe vera juice in a mixing bowl.
2. Add geranium and frankincense essential oils, stirring until well mixed.
3. Use a funnel to transfer the mixture into a glass bottle.
4. Shake before use and apply with a cotton pad after cleansing.

Apple Cider Vinegar and Lavender Toner

This toner combines the purifying qualities of apple cider vinegar with the soothing effects of lavender, helping to tone and balance the skin while minimizing the appearance of pores.

What You Will Need:

- 1/4 cup Apple Cider Vinegar
- 3/4 cup Distilled water
- 8 drops Lavender essential oil
- 5 drops Tea Tree essential oil
- Small mixing bowl
- Measuring cups
- Funnel
- Glass bottle (4 oz.)

What To Do:

1. In a mixing bowl, combine apple cider vinegar and distilled water.
2. Add lavender and tea tree essential oils and mix well.
3. Pour the mixture into the glass bottle using a funnel.
4. Shake before each use and apply to the face with a cotton pad.

Green Tea and Chamomile Toner

This toner blends green tea's antioxidant benefits with chamomile's calming properties, working together to soothe and refresh the skin while reducing redness and irritation.

What You Will Need:

- 1/2 cup Brewed Green Tea (cooled)
- 1/4 cup Chamomile Tea (cooled)
- 10 drops Chamomile essential oil
- 5 drops Lemon essential oil
- Small mixing bowl
- Measuring cups
- Funnel
- Glass bottle (4 oz.)

What To Do:

1. Mix cooled green tea and chamomile tea in a bowl.
2. Add chamomile and lemon essential oils, stirring well.
3. Pour the mixture into a glass bottle using a funnel.
4. Shake well before use and apply with a cotton pad.

Cucumber and Rose Water Toner

This toner combines cucumber's soothing effects with rose water's hydrating properties, helping to calm and replenish the skin while providing a refreshing boost.

What You Will Need:

- 1/2 cup Cucumber juice (freshly made)
- 1/2 cup Rose Water
- 10 drops Rose essential oil
- 5 drops Peppermint essential oil
- Small mixing bowl
- Measuring cups
- Funnel
- Glass bottle (4 oz.)

What To Do:

1. Combine cucumber juice and rose water in a mixing bowl.
2. Add rose and peppermint essential oils, stirring until well blended.
3. Use a funnel to transfer the mixture into a glass bottle.
4. Shake before use and apply with a cotton pad after cleansing.

Aloe and Rosemary Toner

This toner blends the calming properties of aloe with the invigorating benefits of rosemary, designed to soothe and refresh the skin while promoting a balanced complexion.

What You Will Need:

- 1/2 cup Aloe Vera juice
- 1/2 cup Distilled water
- 10 drops Rosemary essential oil
- 5 drops Tea Tree essential oil
- Small mixing bowl
- Measuring cups
- Funnel
- Glass bottle (4 oz.)

What To Do:

1. In a bowl, mix aloe vera juice with distilled water.
2. Add rosemary and tea tree essential oils, stirring well.
3. Pour the mixture into a glass bottle using a funnel.
4. Shake before each use and apply with a cotton pad.

Mint and Lemon Toner

This toner combines the refreshing essence of mint with the brightening properties of lemon, aimed at revitalizing the skin and providing a refreshing, clarifying effect.

What You Will Need:

- 1/2 cup Distilled water
- 1/2 cup Mint Tea (cooled)
- 10 drops Lemon essential oil
- 5 drops Peppermint essential oil
- Small mixing bowl
- Measuring cups
- Funnel
- Glass bottle (4 oz.)

What To Do:

1. Mix distilled water and cooled mint tea in a bowl.
2. Add lemon and peppermint essential oils, stirring until combined.
3. Pour the mixture into a glass bottle using a funnel.
4. Shake before use and apply with a cotton pad.

Orange Blossom and Neroli Toner

This toner blends the soothing properties of orange blossom with the revitalizing essence of neroli, designed to refresh and brighten the skin while providing a calming, uplifting aroma.

What You Will Need:

- 1/2 cup Orange Blossom water
- 1/4 cup Distilled water
- 10 drops Neroli essential oil
- 5 drops Tea Tree essential oil
- Small mixing bowl
- Measuring cups
- Funnel
- Glass bottle (4 oz.)

What To Do:

1. Combine orange blossom water and distilled water in a bowl.
2. Add neroli and tea tree essential oils, stirring well.
3. Use a funnel to pour the mixture into a glass bottle.
4. Shake well before use and apply with a cotton pad.

Witch Hazel and Basil Toner

This toner combines witch hazel's astringent qualities with basil's soothing properties, helping to tighten pores and reduce inflammation while calming and balancing the skin.

What You Will Need:

- 1/2 cup Witch Hazel
- 1/4 cup Distilled water
- 10 drops Basil essential oil
- 5 drops Lavender essential oil
- Small mixing bowl
- Measuring cups
- Funnel
- Glass bottle (4 oz.)

What To Do:

1. Mix witch hazel and distilled water in a bowl.
2. Add basil and lavender essential oils, stirring until well combined.
3. Pour the mixture into a glass bottle using a funnel.
4. Shake before use and apply with a cotton pad.

Cypress and Rose Water Toner

This toner blends cypress's balancing effects with rose water's hydrating properties, designed to regulate oil production and provide a soothing, refreshing finish to the skin.

What You Will Need:

- 1/2 cup Rose Water
- 1/4 cup Distilled water
- 10 drops Cypress essential oil
- 5 drops Lavender essential oil
- Small mixing bowl
- Measuring cups
- Funnel
- Glass bottle (4 oz.)

What To Do:

1. Combine rose water and distilled water in a mixing bowl.
2. Add cypress and lavender essential oils and mix well.
3. Use a funnel to pour the mixture into a glass bottle.
4. Shake well before use and apply with a cotton pad.

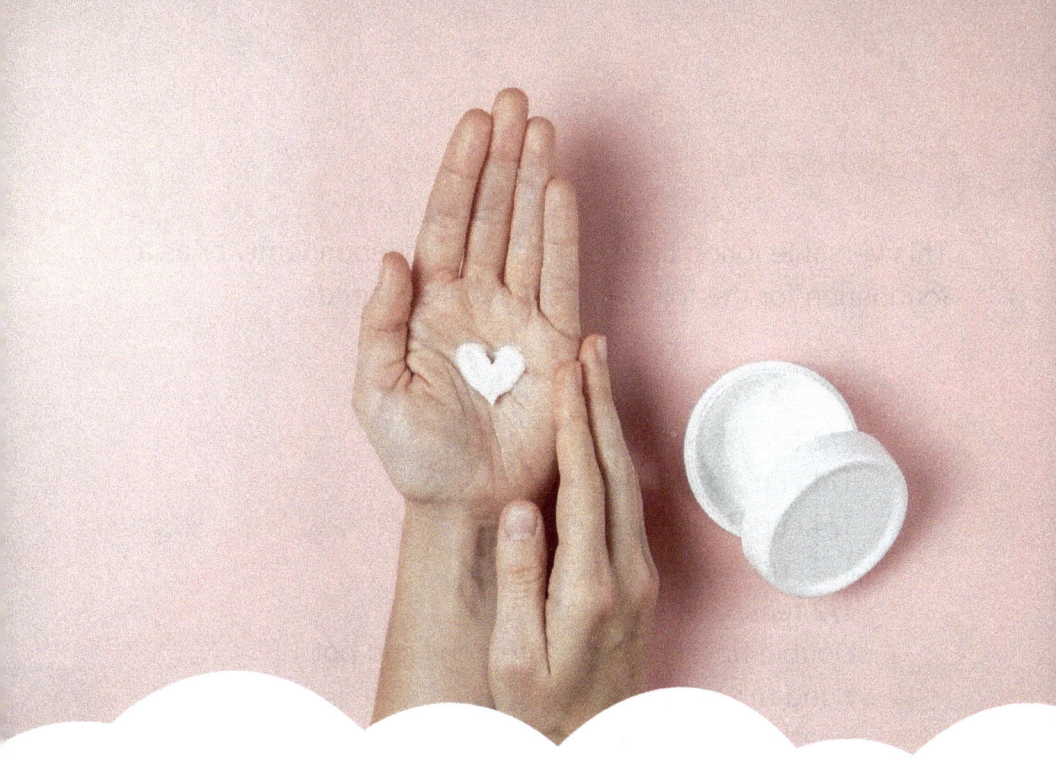

Chapter 22
Moisturizers for Acne

Moisturizers are crucial in any skincare routine, especially for those dealing with acne. While it may seem counterintuitive to moisturize oily or acne-prone skin, the suitable formulation can help balance oil production, soothe inflammation, and maintain the skin's moisture barrier. Essential oils can be powerful allies in these formulations, offering antibacterial, anti-inflammatory, and healing properties. Whether dealing with active breakouts or aiming to prevent future ones, these recipes provide various options to nourish your skin without clogging pores.

Unscented Lotion Base

This versatile lotion base can be used independently or as a foundation for the following essential oil blends.

What You Will Need:

- 1/2 cup Shea Butter
- 1/4 cup Coconut oil
- 1/4 cup Beeswax pellets
- 1/2 cup Aloe Vera gel
- 1/2 teaspoon Vitamin E oil
- Double boiler or heat-safe bowl and pot
- Hand mixer or whisk
- Heat-safe spatula
- Glass jar or lotion bottle for storage

What To Do:

1. Melt shea butter, coconut oil, and beeswax in a double boiler, stirring until entirely melted.
2. Remove from heat and cool slightly before adding aloe vera gel and vitamin E oil.
3. Use a hand mixer or whisk to blend until smooth and creamy.
4. Pour into a glass jar or lotion bottle for storage. Use as a base for the following recipes.

Tea Tree and Lavender Moisturizer

This light moisturizer helps reduce redness and prevent breakouts.

What You Will Need:

- 1/4 cup Unscented lotion base
- 10 drops Tea Tree essential oil
- 5 drops Lavender essential oil
- Small mixing bowl
- Spoon or spatula
- Lotion bottle or jar

What To Do:

1. Combine the unscented lotion base in a small mixing bowl with tea tree and lavender essential oils.
2. Stir until the oils are fully incorporated.
3. Transfer the mixture into a lotion bottle or jar. Apply to clean skin daily.

Aloe and Frankincense Soothing Moisturizer

Perfect for sensitive, acne-prone skin that needs a calming touch.

What You Will Need:

- 1/4 cup Unscented lotion base
- 1 tablespoon Aloe Vera gel
- 8 drops Frankincense essential oil
- 4 drops Roman Chamomile essential oil
- Small mixing bowl
- Spoon or spatula
- Lotion bottle or jar

What To Do:

1. Mix the unscented lotion base with aloe vera gel in a small bowl.
2. Add frankincense and chamomile essential oils and stir well.
3. Pour the mixture into a lotion bottle or jar. Use daily to soothe and hydrate skin.

Mattifying Moisturizer with Geranium and Clary Sage

Controls excess oil production while keeping skin hydrated.

What You Will Need:

- 1/4 cup Unscented lotion base
- 5 drops Geranium essential oil
- 5 drops Clary Sage essential oil
- 1/2 teaspoon Jojoba oil
- Small mixing bowl
- Spoon or spatula
- Lotion bottle or jar

What To Do:

1. Combine the unscented lotion base with geranium and clary sage essential oils in a small mixing bowl.
2. Add jojoba oil and stir until evenly mixed.
3. Transfer the moisturizer into a lotion bottle or jar. Apply to the face after cleansing.

Rosehip and Tea Tree Night Moisturizer

This recipe is designed to help heal acne overnight while nourishing the skin.

What You Will Need:

- 1/4 cup Unscented lotion base
- 10 drops Rosehip Seed oil
- 5 drops Tea Tree essential oil
- 3 drops Lavender essential oil
- Small mixing bowl
- Spoon or spatula
- Lotion bottle or jar

What To Do:

1. Mix the unscented lotion base in a small bowl with rosehip seed oil, tea tree, and lavender oils.
2. Stir until smooth and creamy.
3. Pour into a lotion bottle or jar. Use nightly as part of your skincare routine.

Hydrating Moisturizer with Rose and Chamomile

This provides deep hydration without clogging pores and is ideal for dry, acne-prone skin.

What You Will Need:

- 1/4 cup Unscented lotion base
- 10 drops Rose essential oil
- 5 drops Roman Chamomile essential oil
- Small mixing bowl
- Spoon or spatula
- Lotion bottle or jar

What To Do:

1. Combine the unscented lotion base with rose and chamomile essential oils in a small bowl.
2. Mix until the oils are fully incorporated.
3. Transfer the mixture to a lotion bottle or jar. Apply to the face as needed.

Green Tea and Aloe Moisturizer

Packed with antioxidants, this moisturizer helps calm and protect acne-prone skin.

What You Will Need:

- 1/4 cup Unscented lotion base
- 1 tablespoon Brewed Green Tea (cooled)
- 1 tablespoon Aloe Vera gel
- 5 drops Tea Tree essential oil
- 5 drops Lavender essential oil
- Small mixing bowl
- Spoon or spatula
- Lotion bottle or jar

What To Do:

1. Mix the unscented lotion base with green tea, aloe vera gel, and essential oils in a small bowl.
2. Stir until well combined.
3. Pour into a lotion bottle or jar. Apply daily to help protect and calm the skin.

Chamomile and Calendula Calming Moisturizer

This recipe is ideal for irritated, acne-prone skin that needs extra care.

What You Will Need:

- 1/4 cup Unscented lotion base
- 10 drops Roman Chamomile essential oil
- 5 drops Calendula oil
- Small mixing bowl
- Spoon or spatula
- Lotion bottle or jar

What To Do:

1. Mix the unscented lotion base with chamomile and calendula oils in a small bowl.
2. Stir until thoroughly blended.
3. Transfer to a lotion bottle or jar. Use as needed to soothe and calm the skin.

Neem and Lavender Moisturizer

Neem oil is known for its antibacterial properties, making it an excellent choice for acne-prone skin.

What You Will Need:

- 1/4 cup Unscented lotion base
- 1 teaspoon Neem oil
- 10 drops Lavender essential oil
- Small mixing bowl
- Spoon or spatula
- Lotion bottle or jar

What To Do:

1. Combine the unscented lotion base with neem oil and lavender essential oil in a small bowl.
2. Stir until the oils are fully incorporated.
3. Pour into a lotion bottle or jar. Apply to acne-prone areas as part of your skincare routine.

Aloe Vera and Rosehip Moisturizer

This lightweight moisturizer helps heal and hydrate acne-prone skin.

What You Will Need:

- 1/4 cup Unscented lotion base
- 1 tablespoon Aloe Vera gel
- 10 drops Rosehip Seed oil
- 5 drops Lavender essential oil
- Small mixing bowl
- Spoon or spatula
- Lotion bottle or jar

What To Do:

1. Mix the unscented lotion base in a small bowl with aloe vera gel, rosehip seed oil, and lavender essential oil.
2. Stir until smooth and thoroughly blended.
3. Pour the mixture into a lotion bottle or jar. Apply as needed for hydration and healing.

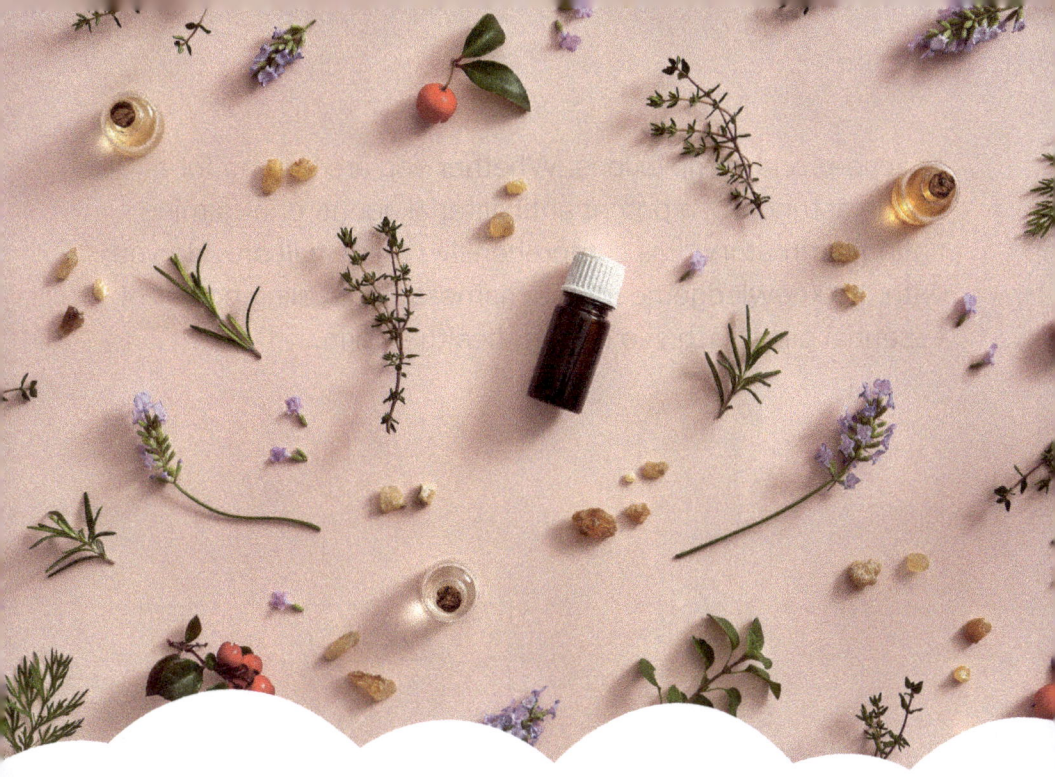

Chapter 23
Essential Oil Directory

This chapter delves into the powerful world of essential oils, focusing specifically on those that have proven benefits for managing and treating acne. The natural potency of essential oils lies in their ability to target the root causes of acne—excess oil production, bacterial infections, inflammation, or scarring. Each oil in this directory has been carefully selected for its unique therapeutic properties that can help clear blemishes, soothe irritated skin, and restore balance to acne-prone complexions. Whether you are looking for a gentle astringent, a potent antibacterial agent, or a calming anti-inflammatory, this comprehensive guide will provide you with the knowledge needed to harness the healing power of essential oils to achieve clearer, healthier skin.

Angelica (Angelica archangelica)

Angelica essential oil is valued for its soothing and anti-inflammatory properties, making it suitable for treating acne and acne-prone skin. It helps to calm irritated skin, reduce redness, and promote the healing of acne breakouts. Angelica oil also has mild astringent properties that help tighten the skin and reduce the appearance of pores, contributing to a clearer complexion. Additionally, its gentle nature makes it suitable for even the most sensitive skin types, helping restore a clear and calm complexion.

Bay (Pimenta racemosa)

Bay essential oil is known for its antibacterial and antiseptic properties, making it effective in treating acne. It helps to cleanse the skin, clear clogged pores, and reduce the occurrence of acne breakouts. Bay oil also has anti-inflammatory effects that help soothe irritated skin and reduce redness and swelling. Its ability to regulate sebum production makes it suitable for oily and acne-prone skin types. Additionally, the warm and spicy scent of Bay can help reduce stress and promote relaxation, which can contribute to clearer skin.

Bay Laurel (Laurus nobilis)

Bay Laurel essential oil is a powerful antiseptic and antibacterial agent, effectively treating acne. It helps to cleanse the skin, clear clogged pores, and reduce the occurrence of acne breakouts. Bay Laurel oil also has anti-inflammatory properties that help soothe irritated skin and reduce redness and swelling. Its ability to regulate sebum production makes it suitable for oily and acne-prone skin types. Additionally, the herbal scent of Bay Laurel can help reduce stress and promote relaxation, which can contribute to clearer skin.

Basil (Ocimum basilicum)

Basil essential oil is renowned for its potent anti-inflammatory and antibacterial properties, making it an excellent choice for treating acne. Its high linalool content helps reduce redness and swelling associated with acne breakouts. Additionally, Basil oil helps purify the skin by eliminating acne-causing bacteria and regulating excess sebum production. Its soothing properties also assist in calming irritated skin, making it suitable for sensitive or inflamed acne-prone areas. Regular use can help clear up existing blemishes and prevent future breakouts, promoting a clearer, healthier complexion.

Benzoin (Styrax benzoin)

Benzoin essential oil is a gentle and soothing remedy for acne-prone skin. Its anti-inflammatory and antibacterial properties help reduce swelling and prevent infections in acne lesions. Benzoin oil also forms a protective layer on the skin, shielding it from environmental pollutants and irritants that can exacerbate acne. Moreover, its warm, resinous aroma has a calming effect, which can help reduce stress-related acne. Regular use of Benzoin oil can promote healing and improve the skin's overall texture.

Bergamot (Citrus bergamia)

Bergamot essential oil is prized for its ability to balance oil production and reduce the appearance of acne. Its antibacterial and antiseptic properties make it effective in preventing the spread of acne-causing bacteria on the skin. Bergamot also has anti-inflammatory effects that help soothe inflamed skin and reduce redness. Additionally, its natural astringent properties help tighten pores and improve skin tone. With its uplifting citrus scent, Bergamot oil can also help alleviate stress, which often contributes to acne breakouts.

Birch (Betula lenta)

Birch essential oil is a natural astringent and antiseptic agent, effectively treating acne. It helps to cleanse the skin, tighten pores, and reduce excess oil production, preventing the formation of acne. Birch oil also has anti-inflammatory properties that help soothe irritated skin and reduce redness. Additionally, its refreshing scent can help uplift the mood and reduce stress, contributing to clearer skin.

Camphor (Cinnamomum camphora)

Camphor essential oil is widely used in treating acne due to its cooling, antiseptic, and anti-inflammatory properties. It helps to soothe inflamed skin, reduce redness, and clear up acne breakouts by eliminating bacteria. Camphor oil also has astringent properties that help tighten the skin and reduce the size of pores, preventing further breakouts. Additionally, its ability to regulate sebum production makes it suitable for oily, acne-prone skin, keeping it balanced and clear.

Cajeput (Melaleuca cajuputi)

Cajeput essential oil is a powerful antiseptic and antibacterial agent that is highly effective in treating acne. It penetrates deeply into the skin to clear clogged pores and eliminate bacteria that cause acne. Cajeput oil also has anti-inflammatory properties, which help reduce the redness and swelling associated with acne breakouts. Additionally, its ability to regulate sebum production can help prevent future breakouts, while its refreshing scent can uplift the mood, helping to alleviate stress-related acne.

Caraway Seed (Carum carvi)

Caraway Seed essential oil is valued for its antibacterial and anti-inflammatory properties, effectively treating acne. It helps to cleanse the skin, clear clogged pores, and reduce the occurrence of acne breakouts. Caraway Seed oil also has astringent effects that help tighten the skin and reduce the appearance of enlarged pores. Its ability to regulate sebum production makes it suitable for oily and acne-prone skin types. Additionally, Caraway Seed's warm and spicy scent can help reduce stress and promote relaxation, contributing to clearer skin.

Carrot Seed (Daucus carota)

Carrot Seed essential oil is valued for its regenerative and healing properties, making it an excellent choice for treating acne and acne scars. Its high content of antioxidants helps repair damaged skin and promotes the growth of healthy new cells. Carrot Seed oil also has anti-inflammatory and antibacterial properties that help reduce acne breakouts and soothe irritated skin. Additionally, it supports detoxification, helping to cleanse the skin and promote a clearer complexion.

Cedarwood (Cedrus atlantica)

Cedarwood essential oil is a natural astringent, making it effective in tightening the skin and reducing the appearance of pores, which can help prevent acne. Its antiseptic properties help cleanse the skin of impurities and eliminate acne-causing bacteria. Cedarwood oil also has anti-inflammatory effects that help soothe irritated skin and reduce the redness and swelling of acne breakouts. Additionally, its ability to regulate sebum production can help keep the skin balanced and prevent future breakouts.

German Chamomile (Matricaria chamomilla)

German Chamomile essential oil is particularly effective in treating inflammatory acne due to its high azulene content. This compound gives the oil its deep blue color and potent anti-inflammatory properties. This oil helps soothe irritated skin, reduce redness, and diminish the appearance of acne scars. Its antibacterial properties also make it effective in preventing new breakouts. German Chamomile is particularly beneficial for individuals with sensitive or reactive skin, providing a calming and healing effect.

Roman Chamomile (Chamaemelum nobile)

Roman Chamomile essential oil is known for its powerful anti-inflammatory and soothing properties, making it ideal for sensitive and acne-prone skin. It helps calm irritated skin, reducing redness and swelling associated with acne. Roman Chamomile also has antibacterial effects that can help prevent acne-causing bacteria from thriving on the skin. Additionally, its gentle nature makes it suitable for even the most sensitive skin types, helping restore a clear and calm complexion.

Cinnamon (Cinnamomum zeylanicum)

Cinnamon essential oil is a powerful antiseptic and antibacterial agent that is highly effective in treating acne. It helps to clear clogged pores, eliminate acne-causing bacteria, and reduce the occurrence of breakouts. Cinnamon oil also has anti-inflammatory properties that help soothe irritated skin and reduce redness and swelling. Its ability to regulate sebum production makes it suitable for oily and acne-prone skin types. Additionally, the warm and spicy scent of Cinnamon can help reduce stress and promote relaxation, which can contribute to clearer skin.

Cistus Labdanum (Cistus ladaniferus)

Cistus Labdanum essential oil is known for its regenerative and anti-inflammatory properties, making it effective in treating acne and acne scars. It helps to promote the healing of acne breakouts and reduce the appearance of scars and blemishes. Cistus Labdanum oil also has astringent effects that help tighten the skin and reduce the appearance of enlarged pores. Its ability to balance sebum production makes it suitable for oily and acne-prone skin types. Additionally, Cistus Labdanum's rich and resinous scent can help reduce stress and promote relaxation, which can contribute to clearer skin.

Citronella (Cymbopogon nardus)

Citronella essential oil is known for its antiseptic and antibacterial properties, making it effective in treating acne. It helps to cleanse the skin, clear clogged pores, and reduce the occurrence of acne breakouts. Citronella oil also has astringent effects that help tighten the skin and reduce the appearance of enlarged pores. Its ability to regulate sebum production makes it suitable for oily and acne-prone skin types. Additionally, Citronella's fresh and uplifting scent can help reduce stress, contributing to clearer skin.

Clary Sage (Salvia sclarea)

Clary Sage essential oil is known for regulating sebum production, making it ideal for balancing oily and acne-prone skin. It has anti-inflammatory and antibacterial properties that help reduce the redness and swelling of acne breakouts while preventing bacterial infections. Clary Sage oil also contains natural phytoestrogens that can help balance hormonal fluctuations, often contributing to acne. Its calming scent can also help reduce stress and anxiety, common acne triggers.

Clove Bud (Syzygium aromaticum)

Clove Bud essential oil is known for its strong antimicrobial and antifungal properties, making it a potent remedy for acne. Its high eugenol content helps eliminate acne-causing bacteria and reduces inflammation in the skin. Clove Bud oil also has analgesic properties that can help relieve the pain associated with severe acne lesions. Additionally, its astringent nature helps tighten the skin and reduce the appearance of enlarged pores, contributing to a clearer complexion.

Coriander (Coriandrum sativum)

Coriander essential oil is known for its antibacterial and antiseptic properties, making it effective in treating acne. It helps to cleanse the skin, clear clogged pores, and reduce the occurrence of acne breakouts. Coriander oil also has anti-inflammatory effects that help soothe irritated skin and reduce redness and swelling. Its ability to control excess oil production makes it suitable for oily and acne-prone skin types, helping to maintain a clear complexion. Coriander's fresh and herbal scent can also help uplift the mood and reduce stress, which can contribute to clearer skin.

Cypress (Cupressus sempervirens)

Cypress essential oil is a powerful astringent that helps tighten the skin and reduce the appearance of pores, effectively preventing acne breakouts. Its antiseptic and antibacterial properties help cleanse the skin and eliminate acne-causing bacteria. Cypress oil also has anti-inflammatory effects that help soothe irritated skin and reduce redness and swelling associated with acne. It also supports circulation, helping promote a healthy and clear complexion.

Eucalyptus (Eucalyptus globulus)

Eucalyptus essential oil is widely used for its potent antibacterial and anti-inflammatory properties, making it effective in treating acne. It helps to cleanse the skin, clear clogged pores, and reduce the occurrence of acne breakouts. Eucalyptus oil also has a cooling effect that soothes irritated skin and reduces redness and swelling. Additionally, its ability to control excess oil production makes it suitable for oily and acne-prone skin types, helping to maintain a clear complexion.

Fleabane (Erigeron canadensis)

Fleabane essential oil is known for its antiseptic and antibacterial properties, making it effective in treating acne. It helps to cleanse the skin, clear clogged pores, and reduce the occurrence of acne breakouts. Fleabane oil also has anti-inflammatory effects that help soothe irritated skin and reduce redness and swelling. Its ability to regulate sebum production makes it suitable for oily and acne-prone skin types. Additionally, Fleabane's fresh and herbal scent can help reduce stress, contributing to clearer skin.

Frankincense (Boswellia carterii)

Frankincense essential oil is revered for its skin-healing properties and is particularly beneficial for acne-prone skin. It has anti-inflammatory and antiseptic properties that help reduce the swelling and redness of acne breakouts while preventing the spread of bacteria. Frankincense oil also promotes cell regeneration, effectively reducing the appearance of acne scars and promoting a more even skin tone. Its calming scent can also help reduce stress, often exacerbating acne.

Galbanum (Ferula galbaniflua)

Galbanum essential oil is known for its potent anti-inflammatory and healing properties, making it effective in treating acne. It helps to soothe irritated skin, reduce redness, and accelerate the healing of acne breakouts. Galbanum oil also has antiseptic properties that help cleanse the skin and prevent bacterial infections that can lead to acne. Additionally, it supports the regeneration of healthy skin cells, helping to reduce the appearance of acne scars and improve skin texture.

Geranium (Pelargonium graveolens)

Geranium essential oil is known for its balancing and healing properties, making it ideal for treating acne. It helps regulate sebum production, preventing excessive oiliness and dryness, which can lead to acne. Geranium oil also has antibacterial and anti-inflammatory effects that help reduce the redness and swelling of acne breakouts. Additionally, it promotes circulation and supports the regeneration of healthy skin cells, helping to fade acne scars and improve overall skin tone. The floral scent of Geranium can also help reduce stress and anxiety, contributing to clearer skin.

Grapefruit (Citrus paradisi)

Grapefruit essential oil is a natural astringent with antibacterial properties, effectively treating acne. It helps to cleanse the skin, tighten pores, and reduce excess oil production, preventing the formation of acne. Grapefruit oil also has anti-inflammatory effects that help soothe irritated skin and reduce redness. Additionally, its high vitamin C content promotes the regeneration of healthy skin cells, helping to fade acne scars and improve skin tone. The refreshing citrus scent of Grapefruit can also help uplift the mood and reduce stress, which can contribute to clearer skin.

Helichrysum (Helichrysum italicum)

Helichrysum essential oil, often called "Immortelle," is highly regarded for its exceptional healing properties, making it a top choice for treating acne and acne scars. It has potent anti-inflammatory, antibacterial, and antifungal properties that help reduce redness, swelling, and the occurrence of acne breakouts. Helichrysum oil also promotes the regeneration of skin tissue, helping to fade acne scars and improve skin texture. Its ability to soothe and heal the skin makes it suitable for all skin types, including sensitive skin.

Hyssop (Hyssopus officinalis)

Hyssop essential oil is a powerful antibacterial and antiseptic agent that is highly effective in treating acne. It helps to clear clogged pores, eliminate acne-causing bacteria, and reduce the occurrence of breakouts. Hyssop oil also has anti-inflammatory properties that help soothe irritated skin and reduce redness and swelling. Its ability to regulate sebum production makes it suitable for oily and acne-prone skin types.

Jasmine (Jasminum officinale)

Jasmine essential oil is known for its soothing and hydrating properties, making it suitable for sensitive and acne-prone skin. It has antibacterial and antiviral effects that help protect the skin from infections and reduce acne breakouts. Jasmine oil also helps regulate oil production, keeping the skin balanced and preventing clogged pores. Its ability to promote skin healing and reduce inflammation effectively treats both active acne and acne scars. Jasmine's sweet and floral aroma can also help uplift the mood and reduce stress, contributing to clearer skin.

Juniper Berry (Juniperus communis)

Juniper Berry essential oil is valued for its detoxifying and cleansing properties, effectively treating acne. It helps to clear clogged pores, eliminate toxins, and reduce the occurrence of acne breakouts. Juniper Berry oil also has astringent properties that help tighten the skin and reduce the appearance of enlarged pores. Its anti-inflammatory effects help soothe irritated skin and reduce redness and swelling associated with acne. Additionally, its ability to regulate sebum production makes it suitable for oily and acne-prone skin.

Lavender (Lavandula angustifolia)

Lavender essential oil is one of the most versatile and widely used oils for treating acne. Its antibacterial and anti-inflammatory properties make it effective in reducing the redness and swelling of acne breakouts while preventing bacterial infections. Lavender oil also promotes the healing of acne scars by encouraging the regeneration of healthy skin cells. Additionally, its soothing properties help calm irritated skin and reduce stress, which can contribute to acne. Lavender is suitable for all skin types and can be used as a spot treatment or added to skincare products for a clearer complexion.

Lemon (Citrus limon)

Lemon essential oil is known for its powerful astringent and antibacterial properties, making it highly effective in treating acne. It helps to cleanse the skin, clear clogged pores, and reduce the occurrence of acne breakouts. Lemon oil also has brightening effects that can help fade acne scars and improve skin tone. Its ability to control excess oil production makes it suitable for oily and acne-prone skin types. In addition, the bright citrus fragrance of Lemon can elevate your mood and relieve stress, which may aid in maintaining healthier skin.

Lemon Myrtle (Backhousia citriodora)

Lemon Myrtle essential oil is a powerful antibacterial and antiseptic agent that is highly effective in treating acne. It helps to clear clogged pores, eliminate acne-causing bacteria, and reduce the occurrence of breakouts. Lemon Myrtle oil also has anti-inflammatory properties that help soothe irritated skin and reduce redness and swelling. Its ability to regulate sebum production makes it suitable for oily and acne-prone skin types. Lemon Myrtle also has antimicrobial and astringent properties that can help cleanse the skin, reduce excess oil, and combat acne-causing bacteria, making it beneficial for maintaining healthy skin.

Lemongrass (Cymbopogon citratus)

Lemongrass essential oil is a powerful astringent and antibacterial agent, effectively treating acne. It helps to cleanse the skin, tighten pores, and reduce excess oil production, preventing the formation of acne. Lemongrass oil also has anti-inflammatory effects that help soothe irritated skin and reduce redness. In addition, the revitalizing citrus scent of Lemongrass can boost the mood and relieve stress, while its antimicrobial and anti-inflammatory properties help cleanse the skin and reduce breakouts, promoting a healthier complexion.

Lime (Citrus aurantiifolia)

Lime essential oil is a natural astringent and antibacterial agent, making it effective in treating acne. It helps to cleanse the skin, tighten pores, and reduce excess oil production, preventing the formation of acne. Lime oil also has brightening effects that can help fade acne scars and improve skin tone. In addition, the zesty and invigorating aroma of Lime can lift the mood and ease stress, while its astringent and antibacterial properties can help reduce excess oil and purify the skin, supporting a clearer complexion.

Linaloe Berry (Bursera delpechiana)

Linaloe Berry essential oil, also known as Mexican Frankincense, is valued for its anti-inflammatory and antiseptic properties, making it effective in treating acne. It helps to reduce redness and swelling while preventing bacterial infections. Linaloe Berry oil also promotes the healing of acne scars by encouraging the regeneration of healthy skin cells. Its soothing properties make it suitable for sensitive and inflamed skin, helping to restore a clear and balanced complexion.

Mandarin (Citrus reticulata)

Mandarin essential oil is a gentle and soothing remedy for acne-prone skin. Its antibacterial and antiseptic properties help prevent the spread of acne-causing bacteria on the skin. Mandarin oil also has anti-inflammatory effects that help reduce redness and swelling associated with acne breakouts. Additionally, its high vitamin C content promotes the regeneration of healthy skin cells, helping to fade acne scars and improve skin tone. In addition, the sweet and uplifting scent of Mandarin can gently nourish and rejuvenate the skin, supporting a more balanced and radiant complexion.

May Chang (Litsea cubeba)

May Chang essential oil, or Litsea Cubeba, is a powerful astringent and antibacterial agent that effectively treats acne. It helps to cleanse the skin, tighten pores, and reduce excess oil production, preventing the formation of acne. May Chang oil also has anti-inflammatory effects that help soothe irritated skin and reduce redness. Additionally, the invigorating aroma of May Chang can help refresh the senses, while its antimicrobial and astringent properties work to balance oily skin and reduce blemishes, contributing to a clearer complexion.

Melissa (Melissa officinalis)

Melissa essential oil, also known as Lemon Balm, is valued for its calming and healing properties, making it suitable for treating acne. It has antibacterial and antiviral effects that help protect the skin from infections and reduce acne breakouts. Melissa oil also has anti-inflammatory properties that help soothe irritated skin and reduce redness and swelling. Its ability to regulate oil production makes it suitable for oily and acne-prone skin types, helping to maintain a clear complexion.

Myrrh (Commiphora myrrha)

Myrrh essential oil has been used for centuries for its healing and regenerative properties, making it an excellent choice for treating acne and acne scars. It has powerful anti-inflammatory and antibacterial effects that help reduce the redness and swelling of acne breakouts while preventing the spread of bacteria. Myrrh oil also promotes skin regeneration, helping to fade acne scars and improve skin texture. Its soothing properties suit all skin types, including sensitive and inflamed skin.

Myrtle (Myrtus communis)

Myrtle essential oil is known for its balancing and healing properties, making it ideal for treating acne. It helps regulate sebum production, preventing excessive oiliness and dryness, which can lead to acne. Myrtle oil also has antibacterial and anti-inflammatory effects that help reduce the redness and swelling of acne breakouts. Additionally, it supports the regeneration of healthy skin cells, helping to fade acne scars and improve overall skin tone.

Neroli (Citrus aurantium var. amara)

Neroli essential oil is prized for its regenerative and healing properties, making it an excellent choice for treating acne and acne scars. It has antibacterial and anti-inflammatory effects that help reduce the redness and swelling of acne breakouts while preventing bacterial infections. Neroli oil also promotes the regeneration of healthy skin cells, helping to fade acne scars and improve skin texture. Its soothing properties suit all skin types, including sensitive and inflamed skin.

Niaouli (Melaleuca quinquenervia)

Niaouli essential oil is a powerful antiseptic and antibacterial agent that is highly effective in treating acne. It penetrates deeply into the skin to clear clogged pores and eliminate bacteria that cause acne. Niaouli oil also has anti-inflammatory properties, which help reduce the redness and swelling associated with acne breakouts. Additionally, its ability to regulate sebum production can help prevent future breakouts, while its refreshing scent can uplift the mood, helping to alleviate stress-related acne.

Opoponax (Commiphora erythraea)

Opoponax essential oil is valued for its soothing and anti-inflammatory properties, making it suitable for treating acne and acne-prone skin. It helps to calm irritated skin, reduce redness, and promote the healing of acne breakouts. Opoponax oil also has mild astringent properties that help tighten the skin and reduce the appearance of pores, contributing to a clearer complexion. Additionally, the warm and resinous scent of Opoponax can provide a calming effect, while its soothing and skin-healing properties help to reduce inflammation and support the regeneration of damaged skin, promoting a more even and healthy complexion.

Orange (Citrus sinensis)

Orange essential oil is a popular choice for treating acne due to its antibacterial and anti-inflammatory properties. It helps to cleanse the skin, clear clogged pores, and reduce the occurrence of acne breakouts. Orange oil also has brightening effects that can help fade acne scars and improve skin tone. With its uplifting citrus aroma, Orange oil helps brighten the skin and its antibacterial properties support a more balanced and radiant complexion.

Oregano (Origanum vulgare)

Oregano essential oil is known for its potent antibacterial and antifungal properties, making it highly effective in treating acne. It helps to cleanse the skin, clear clogged pores, and eliminate acne-causing bacteria, reducing the occurrence of breakouts. Oregano oil also has anti-inflammatory effects that help soothe irritated skin and reduce redness and swelling. Its ability to regulate sebum production makes it suitable for oily and acne-prone skin types. Additionally, the robust and herbal scent of Oregano can help purify the skin with its strong antimicrobial properties, aiding in the reduction of acne and supporting a clearer complexion.

Palmarosa (Cymbopogon martinii)

Palmarosa essential oil is known for its balancing and hydrating properties, making it ideal for treating acne. It helps regulate sebum production, preventing excessive oiliness and dryness, which can lead to acne. Palmarosa oil also has antibacterial and anti-inflammatory effects that help reduce the redness and swelling of acne breakouts. Additionally, it promotes the regeneration of healthy skin cells, helping to fade acne scars and improve overall skin tone. Additionally, the delicate and floral aroma of Palmarosa can help balance the skin's moisture levels, while its antibacterial and hydrating properties support clearer, more youthful-looking skin.

Parsley (Petroselinum crispum)

Parsley essential oil is valued for its antibacterial and anti-inflammatory properties, making it effective in treating acne. It helps to cleanse the skin, clear clogged pores, and reduce the occurrence of acne breakouts. Parsley oil also has astringent effects that help tighten the skin and reduce the appearance of enlarged pores. Its ability to regulate sebum production makes it suitable for oily and acne-prone skin types. Additionally, the fresh and herbal scent of Parsley essential oil can help rejuvenate the skin with its antioxidant and anti-inflammatory properties, which aid in reducing inflammation and promoting a more even, radiant complexion.

Patchouli (Pogostemon cablin)

Patchouli essential oil is known for its anti-inflammatory, antibacterial, and antifungal properties, making it a powerful remedy for acne. It helps to reduce the redness and swelling of acne breakouts while preventing bacterial infections. Patchouli oil also promotes the healing of acne scars by encouraging the regeneration of healthy skin cells. Its moisturizing properties help keep the skin hydrated without clogging pores, making it suitable for all skin types, including oily and acne-prone.

Peppermint (Mentha piperita)

Peppermint essential oil is widely used for its cooling and antibacterial properties, making it effective in treating acne. It helps to cleanse the skin, clear clogged pores, and reduce the occurrence of acne breakouts. Peppermint oil also has anti-inflammatory effects that help soothe irritated skin and reduce redness and swelling. Its ability to control excess oil production makes it suitable for oily and acne-prone skin types, helping to maintain a clear complexion. Additionally, the invigorating and cool aroma of Peppermint essential oil can help refresh and revitalize the skin, while its antimicrobial and astringent properties work to reduce excess oil and soothe inflammation, supporting a clearer complexion.

Petitgrain (Citrus aurantium var. amara)

Petitgrain essential oil is known for its balancing and antiseptic properties, making it effective in treating acne. It helps regulate sebum production, preventing excessive oiliness and dryness, which can lead to acne. Petitgrain oil also has antibacterial and anti-inflammatory effects that help reduce the redness and swelling of acne breakouts. Additionally, it promotes the regeneration of healthy skin cells, helping to fade acne scars and improve overall skin tone. The crisp and woody scent of Petitgrain essential oil can help balance the skin with its astringent and antimicrobial properties, reducing excess oil and blemishes, while promoting a more even and clear complexion.

Plai (Zingiber cassumunar)

Plai essential oil is known for its soothing and anti-inflammatory properties, making it suitable for treating acne and acne-prone skin. It helps to calm irritated skin, reduce redness, and promote the healing of acne breakouts. Plai oil also has mild astringent properties that help tighten the skin and reduce the appearance of pores, contributing to a clearer complexion. Additionally, its gentle nature makes it suitable for even the most sensitive skin types, helping restore a clear and calm complexion.

Rose (Rosa damascena)

Rose essential oil is highly prized for its anti-inflammatory and antibacterial properties, making it effective in treating acne. It helps to reduce redness and swelling while preventing the spread of acne-causing bacteria. Rose oil also has astringent properties that help tighten the skin and reduce the appearance of pores, promoting a smoother complexion. Its ability to hydrate and soothe the skin makes it suitable for sensitive and acne-prone skin. The luxurious and floral aroma of Rose essential oil can help soothe and hydrate the skin, while its anti-inflammatory and regenerative properties support the healing of damaged skin and promote a more balanced and radiant complexion.

Rose Geranium (Pelargonium graveolens)

Rose Geranium essential oil is known for its balancing and regenerative properties, making it effective in treating acne and acne scars. It helps regulate sebum production, preventing excessive oiliness and dryness, which can lead to acne. Rose Geranium oil also has antibacterial and anti-inflammatory effects that help reduce the redness and swelling of acne breakouts. Additionally, it promotes the regeneration of healthy skin cells, helping to fade acne scars and improve overall skin tone. The sweet and floral scent of Rose Geranium essential oil can help balance the skin's oil production and improve its overall tone, while its anti-inflammatory and antimicrobial properties support a clearer, more radiant complexion.

Rosemary (Rosmarinus officinalis)

Rosemary essential oil is widely used for its powerful antiseptic and anti-inflammatory properties, making it effective in treating acne. It helps to cleanse the skin, clear clogged pores, and reduce the occurrence of acne breakouts. Rosemary oil also has astringent properties that help tighten the skin and reduce the appearance of enlarged pores. Its ability to regulate sebum production makes it suitable for oily and acne-prone skin types. Rosemary essential oil, with its herbaceous aroma, can help invigorate the skin. Its antibacterial properties assist in controlling oil production and reducing blemishes, promoting a clearer and healthier complexion.

Rosewood (Aniba rosaeodora)

Rosewood essential oil is known for its regenerative and healing properties, making it an excellent choice for treating acne and acne scars. It has antibacterial and anti-inflammatory effects that help reduce the redness and swelling of acne breakouts while preventing the spread of bacteria. Rosewood oil also promotes the regeneration of healthy skin cells, helping to fade acne scars and improve skin texture. Its gentle nature makes it suitable for all skin types, including sensitive and inflamed skin.

Sage (Salvia officinalis)

Sage essential oil is a powerful antiseptic and anti-inflammatory agent, making it effective in treating acne. It helps to cleanse the skin, clear clogged pores, and reduce the occurrence of acne breakouts. Sage oil also has astringent properties that help tighten the skin and reduce the appearance of enlarged pores. Its ability to regulate sebum production makes it suitable for oily and acne-prone skin types. Additionally, Sage essential oil, with its earthy and herbaceous scent, offers antibacterial benefits that help control acne-causing bacteria and soothe irritated skin, contributing to a clearer and more balanced complexion.

Sandalwood (Santalum album)

Sandalwood essential oil is known for its soothing and anti-inflammatory properties, making it effective in treating acne. It helps to reduce redness and swelling while promoting the healing of acne breakouts. Sandalwood oil also has antibacterial effects that help prevent the spread of acne-causing bacteria. Its ability to hydrate and soothe the skin makes it suitable for sensitive and acne-prone skin. Sandalwood's antimicrobial properties reduce blemishes, promoting a calmer and more even complexion.

Spearmint (Mentha spicata)

Spearmint essential oil is known for its cooling and antibacterial properties, making it effective in treating acne. It helps to cleanse the skin, clear clogged pores, and reduce the occurrence of acne breakouts. Spearmint oil also has anti-inflammatory effects that help soothe irritated skin and reduce redness and swelling. Its ability to control excess oil production makes it suitable for oily and acne-prone skin types, helping to maintain a clear complexion.

Spikenard (Nardostachys jatamansi)

Spikenard essential oil is valued for its soothing and regenerative properties, making it effective in treating acne and acne scars. It has antibacterial and anti-inflammatory effects that help reduce the redness and swelling of acne breakouts while preventing bacterial infections. Spikenard oil also promotes the healing of acne scars by encouraging the regeneration of healthy skin cells. Its calming properties make it suitable for sensitive and inflamed skin, helping to restore a clear and balanced complexion.

Spruce (Picea mariana)

Spruce essential oil is valued for its soothing and anti-inflammatory properties, making it suitable for treating acne and acne-prone skin. It helps to calm irritated skin, reduce redness, and promote the healing of acne breakouts. Spruce oil also has mild astringent properties that help tighten the skin and reduce the appearance of pores, contributing to a clearer complexion. Its balancing properties help regulate oil production, making it beneficial for oily and acne-prone skin, and supporting a clearer complexion.

Tarragon (Artemisia dracunculus)

Tarragon essential oil is known for its anti-inflammatory and antibacterial properties, making it effective in treating acne. It helps to reduce the redness and swelling of acne breakouts while preventing bacterial infections. Tarragon oil also has analgesic properties that can help relieve the pain associated with severe acne lesions. Additionally, its ability to regulate sebum production makes it suitable for oily and acne-prone skin types, contributing to a more even skin tone.

Tea Tree (Melaleuca alternifolia)

Tea Tree essential oil is one of the most popular and effective remedies for acne due to its powerful antibacterial and anti-inflammatory properties. It helps to cleanse the skin, clear clogged pores, and eliminate acne-causing bacteria, reducing the occurrence of breakouts. Tea Tree oil also has astringent effects that help tighten the skin and reduce the appearance of enlarged pores. Its ability to control excess oil production makes it suitable for oily and acne-prone skin types.

Thyme (Thymus vulgaris)

Thyme essential oil is a powerful antibacterial and antiseptic agent that is highly effective in treating acne. It helps to clear clogged pores, eliminate acne-causing bacteria, and reduce the occurrence of breakouts. Thyme oil also has anti-inflammatory properties that help soothe irritated skin and reduce redness and swelling. Its ability to regulate sebum production makes it suitable for oily and acne-prone skin types.

Vetiver (Vetiveria zizanioides)

Vetiver essential oil is known for its soothing and regenerative properties, making it effective in treating acne and acne scars. It has antibacterial and anti-inflammatory effects that help reduce the redness and swelling of acne breakouts while preventing bacterial infections. Vetiver oil also promotes the healing of acne scars by encouraging the regeneration of healthy skin cells. Its grounding and calming properties make it suitable for sensitive and inflamed skin, helping to restore a clear and balanced complexion.

Violet (Viola odorata)

Violet essential oil is valued for its soothing and anti-inflammatory properties, making it suitable for sensitive and acne-prone skin. It helps to calm irritated skin, reduce redness, and promote the healing of acne breakouts. Violet oil also has mild astringent properties that help tighten the skin and reduce the appearance of pores, contributing to a clearer complexion. Additionally, its gentle nature makes it suitable for even the most sensitive skin types, helping restore a clear and calm complexion.

Yarrow (Achillea millefolium)

Yarrow essential oil is known for its soothing and anti-inflammatory properties, making it suitable for treating acne and acne-prone skin. It helps to calm irritated skin, reduce redness, and promote the healing of acne breakouts. Yarrow oil also has mild astringent properties that help tighten the skin and reduce the appearance of pores, contributing to a clearer complexion. Yarrow essential oil, with its calming and anti-inflammatory properties, helps soothe irritated skin and balance oil production, promoting a more even and healthy appearance.

Ylang Ylang (Cananga odorata)

Ylang Ylang essential oil is known for its balancing and soothing properties, making it ideal for treating acne. It helps regulate sebum production, preventing excessive oiliness and dryness, which can lead to acne. Ylang Ylang oil also has antibacterial and anti-inflammatory effects that help reduce the redness and swelling of acne breakouts. Additionally, its calming properties make it suitable for sensitive and inflamed skin, helping to restore a clear and balanced complexion. The sweet and floral scent of Ylang Ylang can also help reduce stress and promote relaxation, which can contribute to clearer skin.

Other Books by
Rebecca Park Totilo

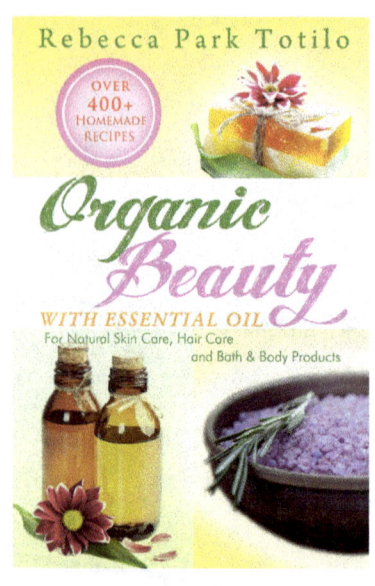

Organic Beauty With Essential Oil: Over 400+ Homemade Recipes for Natural Skin Care, Hair Care and Bath & Body Products

Sweep aside all those harmful chemically-based cosmetics and make your own organic bath and body products at home with the magic of potent essential oils! In this book, you'll find a luxurious array of over 400 eco-friendly recipes that call for breathtaking fragrances and soothing, rich organic ingredients satisfying you head to toe. Included you'll find helpful tips you can have the confidence knowing which essential oil to use and how much when creating your own body scrub, lip butter, or lotion bar! Discover how easy it is to make bath treats like fragrant shower gels, dreamy bubble baths, luscious creams and lotions, deep cleansing masks and facials for literally pennies using essential oils and ingredients from your kitchen.

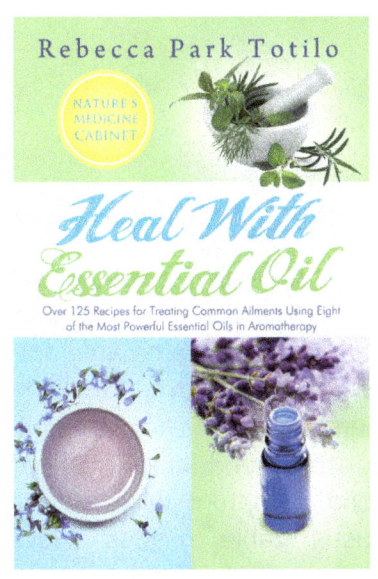

Heal With Essential Oil: Nature's Medicine Cabinet

Using essential oils drawn from nature's own medicine cabinet of flowers, trees, seeds and roots, man can tap into God's healing power to heal oneself from almost any pain. Find relief from many conditions and rejuvenate the body. With over 125 recipes, this practical guide will walk you through in the most easy-to-understand form how to treat common ailments with your essential oils for everyday living. Filled with practical advice on therapeutic blending of oils and safety, a directory of the most effective oils for common ailments and easy to follow remedies chart, and prescriptive blends for aches, pains and sicknesses.

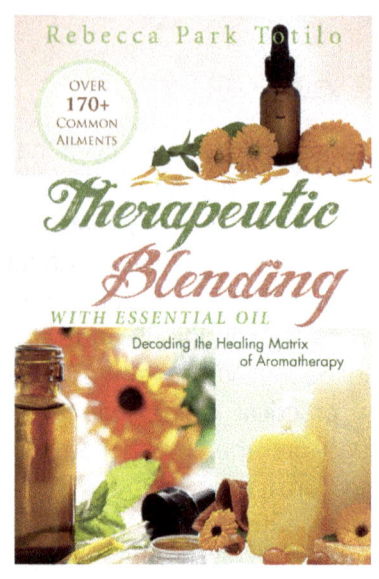

Therapeutic Blending With Essential Oil: Decoding the Healing Matrix of Aromatherapy

Therapeutic Blending With Essential Oil unlocks the healing power of essential oils and guides you through the intricate matrix of aromatherapy, with a compilation of over 170 common ailments. Discover how to properly formulate a blend for any physical or emotional symptom with easy to follow customizable recipes. Now, you can make your own massage oils, hand and body lotions, bath gels, compresses, salve ointments, smelling salts, nasal inhalers and more. This exhaustive guide takes all the guesswork out of blending oils from how many drops to include in a blend, to measuring thick oils, to how often to apply it for acute or chronic conditions. It also shows you how to create a single blend for multiple conditions. Even if you run out of oil for a favorite recipe, this book shows you how to substitute it with another oil.

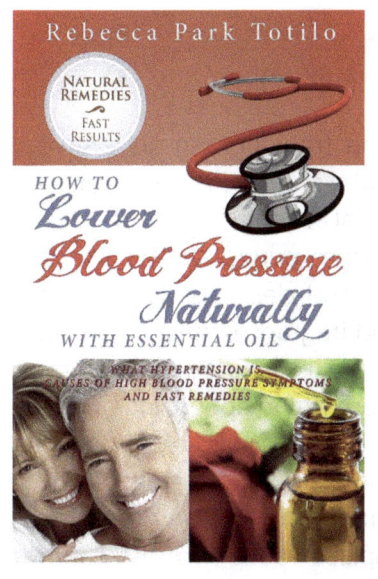

How to Lower Blood Pressure Naturally With Essential Oil: What Hypertension Is, Causes of High Pressure Symptoms and Fast Remedies

One out of three adults have it, and another one-third don't realize it. Oftentimes, it goes undetected for years. Even those who take multiple medications for it still don't have it under control. It's no secret—high blood pressure is rampant in America. High blood pressure, or hypertension, has become a household term. Between balancing meds and monitoring diets though, are the true causes—and best treatments—hidden in the shadows? In How to Lower Blood Pressure Naturally With Essential Oil, Rebecca Park Totilo sheds light on what high blood pressure is, the causes and symptoms of high blood pressure, and which essential oils regulate blood pressure and how to use essential oils as a natural, alternative method.

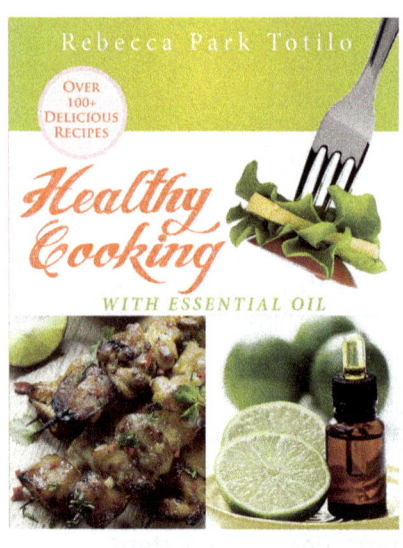

Healthy Cooking With Essential Oil

Imagine transforming an everyday dish into something extraordinary! Essential oils can enliven everything from soups, salads, to main dishes and desserts. Boasting flavor and fragrance, these intense essences can turn a dull, boring meal into something appetizing and delicious. Essential oils are fun, easy-to use and beneficial, compared to the traditional stale, dried herbs and spices found in most pantries today. Healthy food should never be thought of as mere fuel for the body, it should be enjoyed as a multi-sensory experience that brings therapeutic value as well as nourishment. For years we have limited the use of essential oils to scented candles and soaps, in the belief that they were unsafe to consume (and some are!). However, more people are realizing the value of using pure essential oils to enhance their diet. In Healthy Cooking With Essential Oil, you will learn how cooking with essential oils can open up a wealth of creative opportunities in the kitchen.

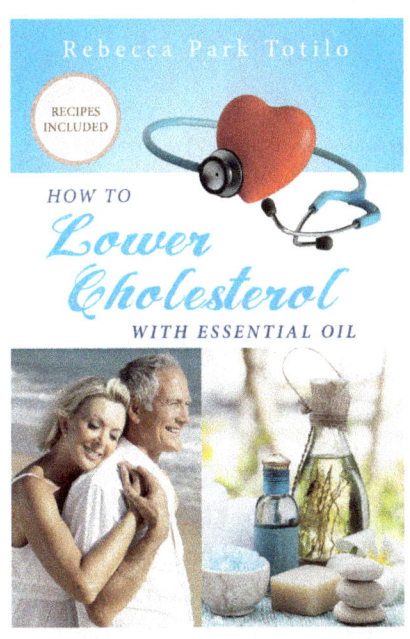

How to Lower Cholesterol With Essential Oil

Take healthy steps now to control high cholesterol and its risk factors with essential oils. People with high cholesterol have twice the risk for heart disease according to the Center for Disease Control and Prevention. What's worse, most folks aren't even aware that they have atherosclerosis until they have a heart attack or stroke. Lowering your cholesterol and triglycerides with essential oils may slow, reduce, or even stop the buildup of dangerous plaque in your arteries causing blockage of blood flow which could result in a heart attack or stroke. In this indispensable guide, author Rebecca Park Totilo presents scientific research supporting the efficacy of certain essential oils for lowering cholesterol, an extensive essential oil and carrier oil directory, natural treatments with recipes, along with easy-to-follow methods of use via inhalation, topically, and ingestion.

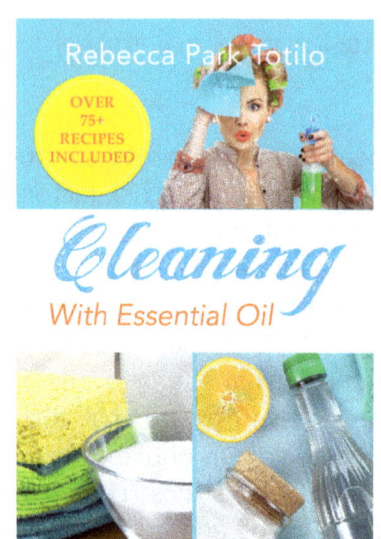

Cleaning With Essential Oil

Now you can have a clean, healthy home free from harsh chemicals using a few ingredients from your pantry and essential oils! Cleaning With Essential Oil features over 75 easy-to-make recipes for every household chore, including laundry detergent, heavy-duty oven cleaner, carpet deodorizer, antibacterial wipes, stain remover, and many more!

Essential oils expert Rebecca Park Totilo guides you in choosing the best essential oils for cleaning based on their chemistry, the health benefits of cleaning with essential oils, and tips for tackling the toughest cleaning jobs from cleaning kitchen appliances to disinfecting bathrooms. The best part is she shows you how to get the entire house clean in less than an hour! Complete shopping lists for supplies and essential oils are provided, so you have everything you need for making your homemade cleaners. Now, you can turn every room into a safe and toxic-free haven for family and pets to enjoy with products like:

- Simple Citrus Soft Scrub
- Stainless Steel Appliance Spray
- Lavender Hand Foaming Soap
- Peppermint Daily Shower Spray
- Minty Fresh Window and Mirror Cleaner
- Garbage Disposal Cleaning Bombs
- Lemon and Geranium Swifty Floor Wipes

In Cleaning With Essential Oil, author Rebecca Park Totilo teaches you how to make your own "green cleaners" without spending a fortune while helping save the planet! Isn't it time you ditch the chemicals and make the switch?

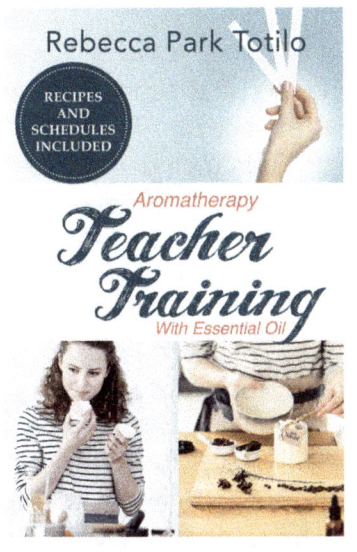

Aromatherapy Teacher Training With Essential Oil

Aromatherapy Teacher Training With Essential Oil provides the essential oil enthusiast the opportunity to craft and hone effective teaching methods for facilitating essential oils classes. This informative book will help you brainstorm and develop unique and interesting aromatherapy workshops, class outlines, and, most importantly, hands-on activities that will keep your students involved and wanting more! Using Rebecca Park Totilo's personal inspirational approach to aromatherapy training, you will come away with the knowledge and confidence to lead and teach your own short workshop or aromatherapy class. Inside this instructional book, you will find:

- The Science of Teaching - Learn how to teach different learning styles, discover your teaching methodology, and develop your own personal techniques for sharing about essential oils.
- The Class - Create a lesson plan from the many themes, choose the best oils to teach, and plan your class with icebreakers, blending projects, venues, and much more.
- Teaching Aromatherapy - Discover how to introduce the safe use of essential oils with detailed step-by-step instructions on demonstrating numerous types of blending projects.
- The Business of Teaching Aromatherapy - Have confidence in knowing what to charge for your classes, develop an elevator speech, and effective marketing for your course.
- Resources - Sample outline and timelines, basic recipes, and a glossary of terms are all included.

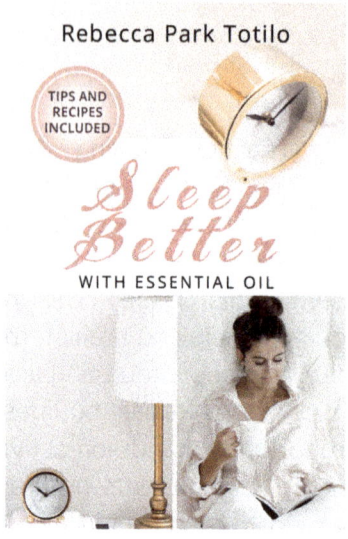

Sleep Better With Essential Oil

It is nighttime, and the sun has disappeared below the horizon. The children are quieting down in their beds, asleep. All the day's chores are done. Text messages and emails have ceased. It is time for sleep. You've changed into your fuzzy pajamas and climbed into a bed with fresh, crisp sheets. You lay your head on a soft pillow and begin to feel your breathing slow down and your eyes grow heavy. In a few short moments, you drift off into a peaceful sleep. The worries of the day vanish, and your mind and body are at rest for the entire night.

This sounds more like a dream for most people. It can be hard to get optimal sleep in this modern age. Some people have trouble sleeping through the night because of things like a crying baby or a toddler who won't go to bed. For others, a busy work schedule and constant notifications on their phone can be distractions. And for some people, there's also the problem of having too much technology available. Social media and TV shows can be so distracting that they make it hard to get enough sleep. Even something as small and seemingly insignificant as drinking caffeine during the day or having a lumpy mattress can prevent restful sleep at night. What are we to do when distractions and outside forces steal our sleep?

Fortunately, there is hope for those struggling to get quality, consistent sleep. Hundreds of thousands of people worldwide have discovered the potent nature of essential oils to create a restful environment in their homes every night. The aroma of these oils can be combined with other healthy practices before bedtime for an even better experience. This book touches on some important aspects of sleeplessness and essential oils. Hopefully, it will answer questions you have on how to use essential oils at bedtime and create a more restful environment for getting the best sleep possible.

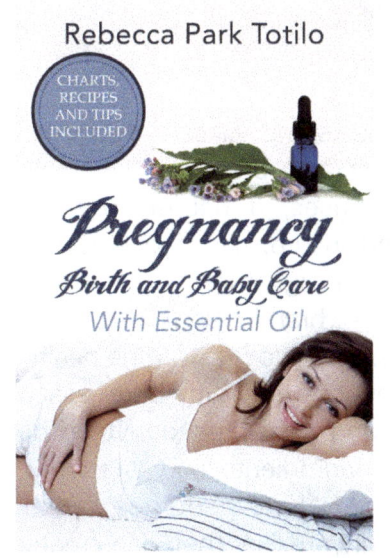

Pregnancy, Birth, and Baby Care With Essential Oil

Pregnancy, Birth, and Baby Care With Essential Oil shows you how to safely use essential oils for all types of issues that arise during pregnancy, labor, and postpartum. Unlike traditional pregnancy guidebooks that follow conventional, fear-based instruction, this book offers a healthy approach to pregnancy, childbirth, and baby care, embracing a natural and safe way to use essential oils.

Full of advice and tips for a healthy pregnancy, Rebecca Park Totilo's researched-based remedies for common and troublesome symptoms guide you with the utmost care given to the health of you and your unborn child.

- Safe and Effective Essential Oils Treatments that address a range of ailments and concerns before and after the baby arrives. Details over 50 different pregnancy discomforts and challenges from morning sickness to insomnia, acne to backaches, heartburn to stretchmarks - and how aromatherapy can help.
- Numerous Charts outline specific essential oils safe for use during pregnancy, labor and delivery, nursing, and newborn care
- Detailed Profiles of 45 Essential Oils provides a comprehensive understanding of the medicinal properties, chemical makeup, and precautions of each essential oil.
- Over 100+ Essential Oils Recipes professionally formulated with step by step instructions for use in the bath, in a massage, and for diffusing around your home.

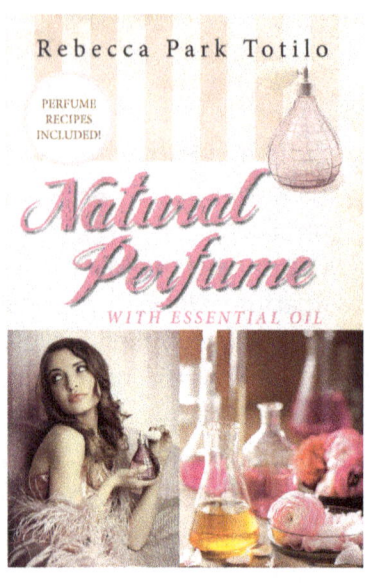

Natural Perfume With Essential Oil

Using the same classic perfumery techniques and processes as mainstream houses, a natural perfumer can blend, dilute, age and bottle his or her own signature scent, rivaling any name brand. Perfumes, body splashes, and colognes can be healthy too when created with pure essential oils and absolutes derived from botanical ingredients harvested from the earth. Natural perfumes can be eco-friendly, unlike their lab-created synthetic counterparts whose chemicals are considered toxic environmental hazards. Now you can create natural fragrances that are subtle, giving you an aura of sweet bliss within your breathing space—only a few feet from your body. When you leave the room, your fragrance goes with you. In this guide, you will discover how to create natural Eau de parfums that develop in layers, changing gradually with the chemistry of your skin. Working in unison with your body's chemistry, your fragrance gently evolves into your own signature scent, so you smell like you, not like everybody else. Discover how to create unique fragrances unlike anything on the market that will captivate your senses.

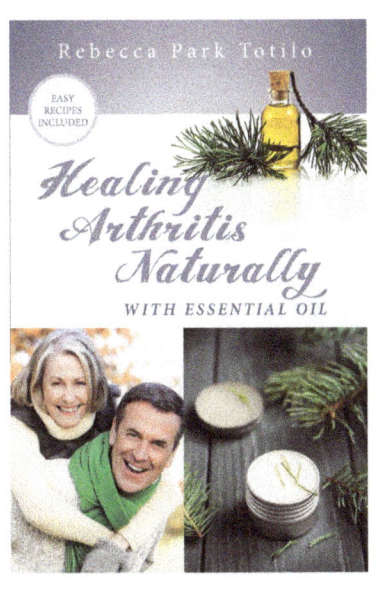

Healing Arthritis Naturally With Essential Oil

If you feel a bit like the tin man in the Wizard of Oz because your joints creak or don't move when you want them to, maybe they are asking you for oil - essential oils that is. Why live with pain or limited mobility if you don't have to? Medical research provides compelling evidence that essential oils can relieve pain and inflammation whether its due to a sports injury or arthritis, and offers the least invasive orthopedic treatment available. As the leading cause of disability in America today and the most common chronic disease to affect those over the age of 40, arthritis comes in over 100 different forms, and all share one main characteristic: joint inflammation. If you're one of the 50 million worldwide affected by arthritis, nature has provided a remedy. In this book, author Rebecca Park Totilo shares valuable information on the causes and symptoms of arthritis and how to use essential oils as a natural alternative. Discover which essential oils reduce inflammation and pain and how to formulate blends using essential oils. You will find dozens of recipes for lotions, salves, bath salts, and more in this how-to guide!

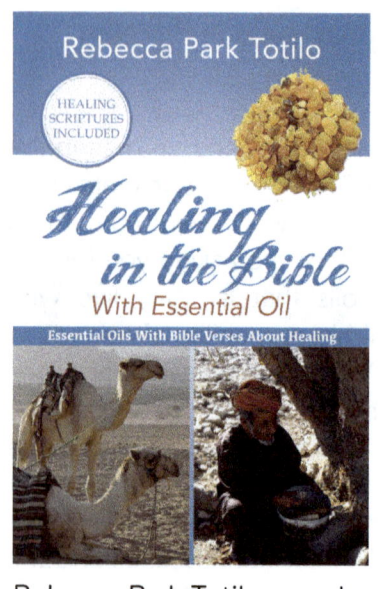

Healing in the Bible With Essential Oil

Since the creation, essential oils have been inhaled, applied to the body, and taken internally in which the benefits extended to every aspect of their being. Buried within the passages of scriptures lies a hidden treasure - possibly every man's answer to illness and disease. Now you can learn their secrets and discover how to transform your life and walk in divine health. In this book, Healing in the Bible With Essential Oil, Certified Aromatherapist Rebecca Park Totilo reveals various aspects of every fragrance mentioned in the Bible.

You will discover each essential oil:

- Rich biblical history and/or pagan roots
- Spiritual significance, symbolism, and hidden meaning
- Healing properties, including traditional uses, medicinal properties, and applications
- Scripture references, Hebrew or Greek meanings, and usage
- Rituals and recipes for making holy water, anointing oil, healing salves, and incense

Based on science and research, over 30 essential oil datasheets are included showing the breakdown of the chemical components, helping you to identify the oil's therapeutic benefits with safety information.

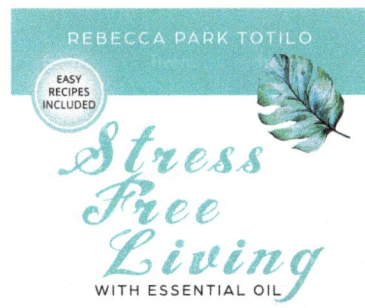

Stress Free Living With Essential Oil

Everyone experiences stress from time to time. But when stress goes unchecked over time, it can play havoc on a person's health. Chronic stress results in a complete breakdown of the body and mental health. In Stress-Free Living With Essential Oil, author Rebecca Park Totilo offers a natural solution for handling the symptoms of stress using essential oils.

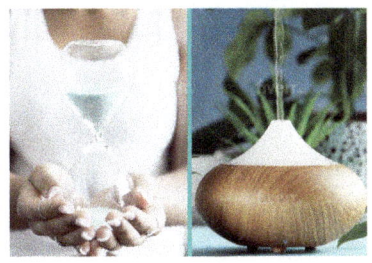

Based on scientific studies, Rebecca lists which essential oils can effectively reprogram the stress response on a chemical level in the brain and interrupt unhealthy stress responses - quickly shifting the body towards homeostasis. Discover how to live a stress-free life using essential oils. Numerous recipes and tips are included in this how-to guide!

www.ingramcontent.com/pod-product-compliance
Lightning Source LLC
Chambersburg PA
CBHW070635160426
43194CB00009B/1468